NAIL
IT!

To my family – Dad, Katy and Grandad, but especially to my Mum,
my inspiration, without whose help and encouragement this book
wouldn't have been possible.

THIS IS A CARLTON BOOK

Published in 2015 by Carlton Books Limited
20 Mortimer Street
London W1T 3JW

10 9 8 7 6 5 4 3 2 1

A CIP catalogue record for this book is available from the British Library.

ISBN 978 1 78097 625 9

Senior Executive Editor: Lisa Dyer
Managing Art Director: Lucy Coley
Designer: Emma Wicks
Production Manager: Maria Petalidou
Cover by Lucy Coley

Printed in Dubai

NAIL IT!

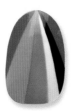

Sophie Harris-Greenslade

CARLTON BOOKS

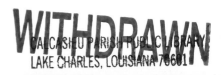

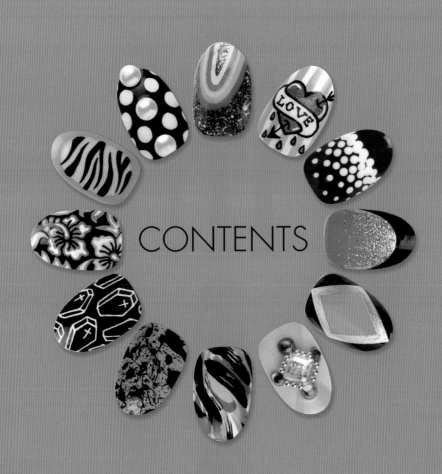

CONTENTS

INTRODUCTION

Nail art is everywhere! From the catwalk to fashion campaigns, on celebrities, on the high street and even in exhibitions.

It's an artistic, fun form of self expression, enjoyed worldwide by the young and mature alike. Nail art has become an affordable, accessible luxury that everyone can partake in, whether at the salon or at home. There is no doubt about it – nail art has become the ultimate fashionable creative outlet and a must-have accessory!

Nail art, however, is not new. It's been around since ancient times. It is said to have originated in India in 5,000 BC, when women used to dye their nails with henna. Throughout history, various peoples and cultures have adorned their nails to indicate wealth and social status.

In recent years nail art has seen a phenomenal surge in popularity. With new technology, brands have been busy creating and developing a variety of innovative nail polishes, effects and textures. This has helped assist the nail artist with their professional development as well as feeding the ever-growing demand for DIY nail art. New techniques and styles are always evolving, with technology creating products to keep us ever excited and experimental when it comes to our nail art. There is such a variety of shades and innovative effect polishes as well as nail art pens, embellishments, foils and kits that you can purchase to experiment with at home. The possibilities are endless!

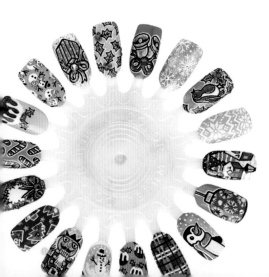

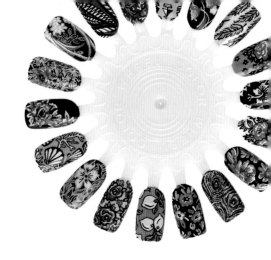

I have been around nail art nearly all my life thanks to my nail artist mother, who has been in the beauty industry for over twenty years. When I was younger she painted Union Jack nails for me to go to a Spice Girls concert and I would sit and paint false nail tips for fun with her at home! I initially trained as an illustrator but my love for art and design and nail art seemed to go hand in hand. As a result I went on to study manicure, pedicure and nail technology and work in salons in London.

The rise in the popularity of nail art led my blog , The Illustrated Nail, to gain a huge worldwide following. These days I mainly work as a session nail stylist on editorial and advertising shoots as well as working for numerous fashion and beauty brands on a variety of projects around the world including OPI and Christian Dior. I am lucky enough to have worked at London Fashion Week for designers such as Jasper Conran, Daks, Matthew Williamson and PPQ as well as on editorial shoots for *Tatler, Vanity Fair* and *Vogue*.

In this book you'll find over 100 fashion-forward nail designs for every occasion. Each design has detailed step-by-step instructions as well as top tips and advice on technique, materials and tools. From simple, classic designs such as houndstooth and half-moons to more intricate batik and tribal designs, there is something for everyone, from the novice nail art beginner to the professional session nail tech. You'll also find a chapter full of striking styles inspired by, and perfect for, fashion shoots and catwalk shows.

Throughout the book you'll learn how to create a range of effects and techniques including water marbling, dotting, splatter and ombré nails. You can create any of the designs on natural nails, press-ons or nail enhancements – the designs can be adapted for all shapes and nail sizes. The techniques and tips you'll learn throughout the book will, I hope, help you not only to copy the designs here, but also to experiment and create your own stand-out nail art.

Sophie Harris-Greenslade

HAND AND NAIL CARE

Caring well for the hands and nails will help you avoid problems as well as prevent premature ageing. Regular manicures maintain the condition of skin and nails. Between manicures, keep your skin moisturized and use sun screen protection. Avoid using your nails as tools, as this leads to breakage and damage. When carrying out household chores, wear gloves, particularly if washing dishes, as liquid detergents can strip the hands and nails of moisture.

NAIL HEALTH AND GROWTH

Fingernails are made of keratin, the same protein from which our hair is made. Healthy nails should be smooth with no discolouration. The nail plate is formed of layers with minimal moisture and oil content cementing the layers together. As such, you should avoid soaking your nails in water. Although this is sometimes done at the salon for a pampering experience, it's actually better to perform a dry manicure. Water dries out the nails, leaving them weak, brittle and prone to breaking.

CUTICLE HEALTH

Don't cut or remove your cuticles – they're there for a reason! They prevent bacteria from entering the nail fold and protect the "matrix", which is the area where the nail cells grow. Removing the cuticle means it will grow back thicker in response to the damage. Always use cuticle oil,

especially in colder weather when our skin can become dryer. Apply once a day after you have a shower or before you go to bed. Keep cuticles in shape by teasing them back after a shower with either your finger wrapped in a towel or tissue, with a metal or plastic cuticle tool or with a cuticle stick tipped with cotton.

Choose a good-quality cuticle oil, such as almond oil. If you tend to pick at your cuticles, using an oil regularly will stop them from becoming dry so there'll be nothing to pick at!

TROUBLESHOOTING PROBLEMS

A healthy nail can reflect the health of the person. A great nail design will benefit from a healthy, smooth nail plate, so it is important to recognize problems to be able to prevent, treat or fix them. Here are a few problems you may encounter.

Ridges

These are longitudinal grooves or furrows along the length of the nail plate. Ridges can be shallow or deep and may be caused by trauma, mechanical or physical damage such as removing enhancements incorrectly, or by ageing. Regular manicures including buffing, which will exfoliate the nail plate, will help minimize ridges. A ridge filler or ridge-filling base coat will help smooth out the nail plate.

Weak and Brittle Nails

These are nails that break easily, often below the free edge. Clients with weak, brittle nails

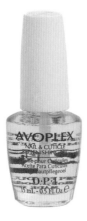
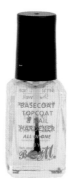
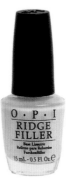
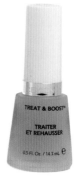

cannot usually grow them to a good length. This condition can be caused by neglect, particularly by not using gloves when washing dishes. Regular dry manicures including oil treatments will help improve the condition and hand cream and cuticle oil should be used frequently. A nail-strengthening product should also be used.

Split Nails

These are nails prone to splitting down the length of the nail, usually starting at the tip and extending towards the cuticle. Lack of moisture and oil is usually the cause and the solution is the same for weak nails, above. You can also apply an overlay to add protection.

Peeling Nails

The nail plate consists of layers cemented together with moisture and oil. When moisture or oil is lost from the nail plate, it is then prone to peeling. This can occur because of regular, prolonged immersion in water. If you cannot avoid this, use nail strengtheners or overlay and

apply a barrier cream regularly. The solution is the same as for weak and brittle nails.

White Spots

Also known as leukonychia, white spots were once thought to be caused by a lack of calcium or zinc. Now the cause is considered to be minor trauma to the nail as it is forming in the matrix; as the nail grows, the trauma is seen in the nail plate. The spots are harmless and nail art and polish will help disguise the condition.

Hangnail

A hangnail is a small, torn piece of hard skin or cuticle at the sides of the nails. Pulling off the hangnail will be painful and may lead to infection. Regular manicures will prevent hangnails occurring, as will regular use of hand cream and cuticle oil. Nail biters are prone to hangnails, as they have their nails in their mouth, which dries out the skin. Cuticle nippers can be used to remove the hangnail, cutting as close to the skin as possible.

MY ESSENTIAL MANICURE KIT

Everyone's manicure kit will differ, as each person will have specific preferences on tools and products. My personal essential manicure kit consists of the following:

I Hand Sanitizer

A good-quality, antibacterial hand sanitizer should be used to cleanse the hands and nails prior to carrying out a manicure or nail art design. It is important as it protects the client and anyone in the workplace. The most common forms are sprays or wipes.

2 Nail Files

A fine grit emery file or a glass file should be used on natural nails to refine nail edges and create shape. Although glass files can be more expensive, they are best for preventing splitting and peeling. They also last longer than emery files and can be effectively sanitized. Files are graded by grit: the lower the number, the coarser the file. For natural nails use one with a grit of 240 upwards – anything below that is best for nail enhancements.

3 Four-Way Buffer

This is a four-sided combination file-and-buffer that exfoliates, buffs and polishes the natural nail, ultimately producing a high shine on the nail plate. It also stimulates circulation, which will improve the health of the nail.

4 Cuticle Remover

Cuticle remover is used to remove the dead cuticle that has adhered to the nail plate. It is

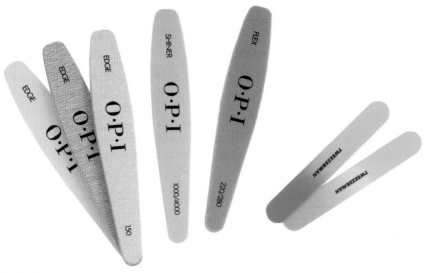

a caustic product so should be used with care: avoid contact with the skin and apply to the cuticle and nail plate only, using a cotton bud. Follow manufacturer's instructions for use as products do differ in their application.

5 Cuticle Pusher

A cuticle pusher or dual tool is a specialized metal implement which is used to ease back the cuticle and remove dead cuticle that has adhered to the nail plate. Good-quality, surgical stainless-steel implements should be used. For home use, you can tease back cuticles with a plastic cuticle stick.

6 Cuticle Nippers

This small, specialized tool is used to remove hangnails and any ragged cuticles. You should not remove live cuticle. Use good-quality nippers made of surgical stainless steel.

7 Cuticle Oil

Used to soften and nourish the cuticles, choose one that contains oils such as jojoba, almond or vitamin E. Cuticle oil can be used as frequently as required by applying a small amount and massaging in with small circular movement around the cuticle. Those who have nut allergies must avoid nut oils.

8 Base Coat

Applied prior to nail colour, a base coat protects the nail plate and acts as an anchor for the polish in order to extend longevity. It is also used to prevent coloured polish from staining the nail plate. You can also buy ridge-

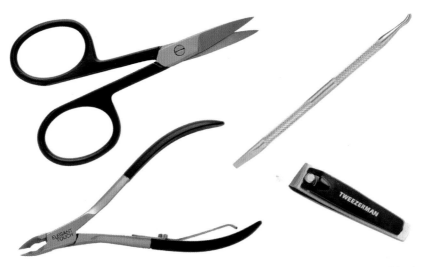

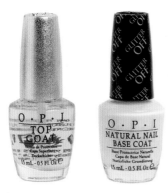

be used with lint-free pads with individual ones used for red and very dark colours to avoid spreading the pigment to other nails and skin. Soak the pad in remover and place onto the nail for a few seconds, allowing the solvent to dissolve the polish, then wipe away from the cuticle with a firm stroke. Repeat as necessary. If removing nail polish from enhancements, avoid acetone-based removers as it may compromise the enhancement.

12 Lint-free Pads
Whenever possible, use lint-free pads as regular cotton wool has fibres that can spoil your polish and design.

13 Nail Treatments
There are a few nail and skin conditions that require additional products. If a client has weak, brittle or split nails, a nail strengthener or hardener can be incorporated into the manicure to protect and strengthen the nail plate. For those with ridges, grooves or furrows, a ridge filler or ridge-filling base coat can be used.

MY ESSENTIAL NAIL ART KIT
See also pages 18-29.

1   Nail Art Pens
2   Fine Artist Brushes
3   Striping Brush
4   Dotting Tool
5   Tidy-up Brush

filling base coats that will fill in ridges, thus ensuring an even finish.

9 Top Coat
The final stage application, a top coat provides a high-gloss shine, protects the polish from chipping and extends the longevity of the colour. It is also used for nail art when sealing acrylic paint or embellishments such as gems, bullion beads, etc.

10 Hand Cream
Hand cream or lotion is essential to moisturize the hands and cuticles. Generally, cream is used for very dry or mature hands and lotion is for normal skin, as its formulation is lighter in texture with less oil content. Apply frequently with small circular massaging movements.

11 Nail Polish Remover
Nail polish remover is a solvent that dissolves polish, removing it from the nail plate. It should

CARING FOR YOUR TOOLS AND PRODUCTS

Always sanitize and sterilize your tools before and after use. For professional technicians, there are various sterilization methods to choose from, such as autoclave, bead sterilizer, chemical, etc. For home use, a chemical bath is the most common. First wash your brushes and tools using soap and hot water to remove any debris. Then place tools in the chemical bath following the manufacturer's instructions. Some brushes cannot be submerged, therefore need to be wiped over with an antibacterial cleansing product. Sanitizing working surfaces and products can be carried out using an antibacterial sanitizing spray and wiping clean with disposable towels. This should be done before and after every client to prevent cross-contamination.

• Store sterilized products and tools in clean airtight containers between uses.

• Keep polishes out of direct sunlight.

• Over time polish can build up around the neck of the bottle and prevent the lid from closing, meaning the polish inside will be exposed to the air and the solvents in it will evaporate. This is what makes the polish go thick and gloopy! To keep your polishes in tip-top condition, wipe the bottle neck clean every time you use the polish, using a little nail polish remover on a lint-free pad.

• If your polishes have already gone a little thick and are difficult to use, use nail polish thinner to restore them; this is specially formulated to thin and prolong the life of your polish.

• Avoid using nail polish remover to thin polish as, in the long run, it will make things worse! It generally contains additives like perfume and oils that are not found in nail polish, so adding these can cause colour to separate and break down.

• Where possible use disposable items (emery boards, etc) to avoid cross-contamination.

• Check the quality of tools regularly. Broken or worn-out tools should be replaced.

THE BASIC MANICURE

Preparation is important prior to nail art application to ensure longevity of the design. A mini dry manicure should be carried out where possible. This should include sanitizing, easing back of the cuticles, removing any excess cuticle that has adhered to the nail plate, filing the nails to shape, buffing to remove surface shine, dehydration and application of a base coat. Follow these simple steps below.

1 Sanitize

Using an antibacterial spray, wipes or gel, wipe over the hands to remove any dirt or oil. Check the hands and nails for any problems, conditions or contraindications (look for anything that prevents you carrying out the manicure or nail art).

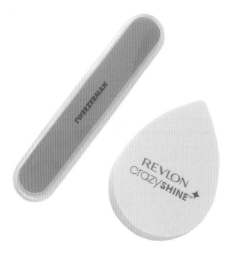

2 Decide on Your Nail Shape

There is no right or wrong when it comes to nail shape as it all falls down to preference, lifestyle and current fashion trends. However a general rule for natural nails is to mirror the natural shape of the cuticle line.

There are five basic nail shapes: oval, square, squoval, round and almond/pointy, but new shapes including stiletto and coffin have also recently become popular. The best shape to prevent breakages is squoval and is perfect for natural shorter nails. Oval and almond are classic flattering shapes, perfect for wide, narrow, short or long. With nail enhancements you can enjoy any shape you like as the overlay increases the strength.

3 Shape Your Nails

Choosing the appropriate file for either natural nails or enhancements, file to refine or shape your nails. At one time, filing with a see-saw motion was frowned upon, as it was thought to cause weak and brittle nails. The damage, however, was caused by coarse emery boards of poor quality. Glass files are of superior quality with a much finer grit and do not cause this problem so you can file back and forth, if desired.

4 Cuticle Work

To remove dead cuticle, first apply cuticle remover to the cuticle and nail plate using a cotton bud. Using a cuticle pusher/dual tool, gently ease back the cuticles while removing dead cuticle from the nail plate. Wipe debris onto a clean tissue.

5 Moisturize

Apply hand cream or lotion to the hand and cuticles using small circular massage movements. If you are working on someone else and the product is cold, warm it first by massaging it in your own hands.

6 Buffing

Buffing the nails every one to two weeks stimulates blood circulation, which can improve the health of the nail and promote growth. Avoid overbuffing however, as this can thin the nail plate, causing nails to become weak. Overbuffing creates friction, which creates heat, and heat will dry out the nail plate, making it susceptible to becoming weak and brittle.

Use the four-way buffer using the coarsest grit first, working through to the shine buffer. A little oil can be used at the final buffing stage to maximize shine.

If applying polish, it is not necessary to buff to a shine. Use the coarser side of the buffer to lightly etch the nail plate, removing surface shine and any oils that can prevent good adhesion of the polish.

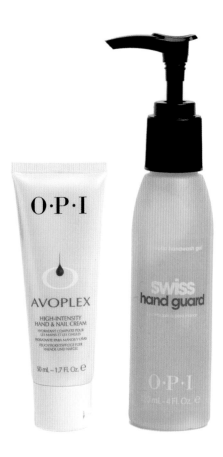

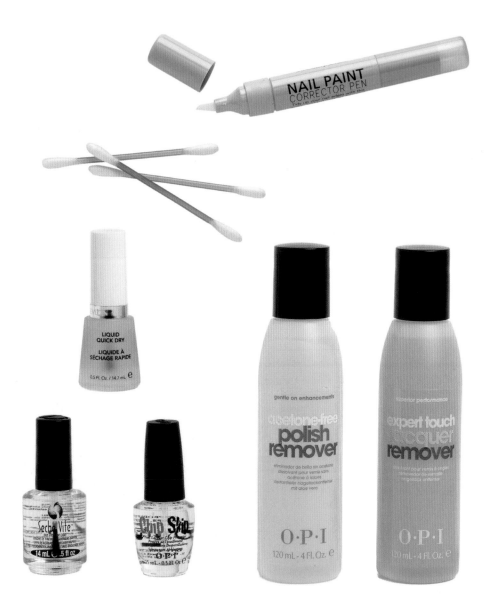

POLISH PREP & CLEAN UP

After your manicure (see pages 14–15) and before applying polish, always "squeak" the nail by using a lint-free pad soaked in remover to wipe over the nail. This gets rid of any dust or debris and any naturally occurring oils on the surface of the nail plate that prevent the polish from adhering and so cause it to chip. It is a great technique for extending the length of your manicure!

Base Coat

When working on natural nails always use a good base; a base coat will prevent discolouration, minimize any ridges in the nail plate, act as an anchor to ensure good adhesion of polish and will prolong the longevity of the nail art design.

Finishes

To get that super shiny salon effect and to prevent your manicure from premature chipping finish off with a good quality top coat.

Quick-dry Top Coat/Quick-dry Drops

Use a quick-dry top coat or quick-dry drops to seal in your manicure. Paint all layers of polish as thinly as possible so that they dry more quickly, thus preventing smudging.

Clean Up

Use either nail corrector pens or a brush dipped in acetone/nail polish remover to correct any mistakes. Avoid using wooden sticks tipped with cotton as the cotton fibres get stuck in the polish! Most good nail companies produce specially formulated nail polish corrector products.

Removing Polish

When removing polish, avoid rubbing the colour all around the finger. Soak a lint-free pad in nail polish remover and hold onto the nail for a few seconds so that the polish remover has time to penetrate and soften the polish. Then swipe the cotton pad away from the cuticle and most of the polish should come off in one clean motion. When removing really dark polish, particularly red, use a new pad for each finger, otherwise the polish on the pad will transfer to the next finger.

ADVICE FOR PROFESSIONALS

Professionals should always follow relevant legislation depending on where you live, such as the Health & Safety at Work Act and Control of Substances Hazardous to Health (COSHH) in the UK and the Environmental Protection Agency (EPA) in the USA. As a trained professional it is important to ensure that you comply with current as well as any new legislation and codes of practice. This will protect you, the client and any work colleagues. In the UK, the Hairdressing and Beauty Industry Authority (HABIA) is the standards setting body for nail services (please refer to the Code of Practice for Nail Services at www.habia.org).

NAIL ART TOOLS

BRUSHES

Brushes are available in various types and sizes, and come in a variety of hairs, including synthetic, nylon and sable. The brush you use will depend on the design and effect you want to achieve so try out different types to find which one suits you best.

Fine Detail Brush

This is generally the smallest and finest of the brushes and is used for very finely detailed designs.

Striping Brush

A long and thin brush, this is generally used for line work and is perfect for painting stripes. It is available in different widths and lengths and can be made from either natural hair or manmade fibres. Super stripers have extra long, thin hairs and are used for wisps and flicks.

Striping Brush in a Bottle

Available in a range of colours, these are polishes that contain a striping brush. They can also be purchased empty so that you can fill the bottle with polish remover and use the brush to dip into any of your polish colours. The remover inside the bottle cleans the brush between colour changes, but the bottle must be cleaned and the remover changed regularly.

Fan Brush

Used to create texture and blend colours together, it can also be used to smooth on gold or silver leaf.

Dusting Brush

This is used as a tidy brush for non-wet products, such as glitter and coloured dust.

Tidy-up Brush

Dip into polish remover and use to clear away those tiny amounts of stray colour.

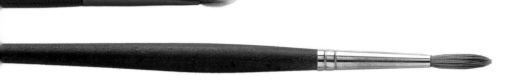

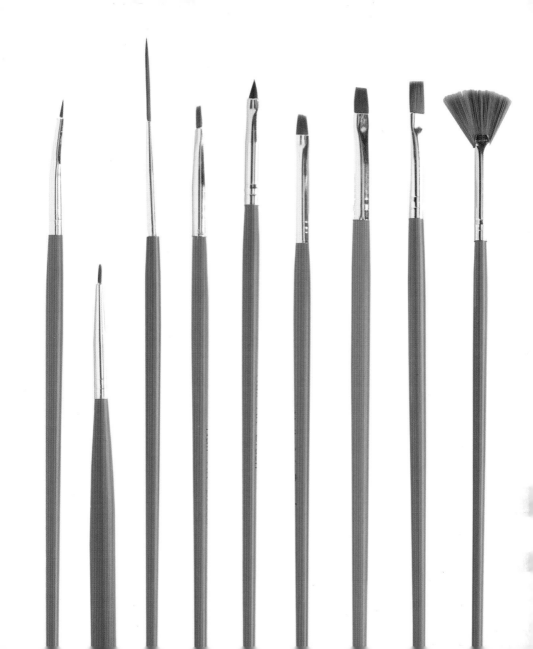

NAIL ART PENS

Used to create intricate nail art designs, nail art pens contain polish that is generally of a thinner consistency, as the polish needs to pass through the tiny nib. They are available in "felt-tip" versions that need to be applied to a dry surface and nibbed versions that need to be squeezed to release the polish. Drawing with them tends to be tricky to master, but they are extremely versatile as they can be used to create a number of effects from fine details to lines, swirls and dots.

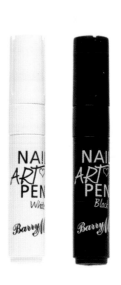

- To use, first squeeze a little of the polish out onto tissue to get rid of any blockages or air bubbles that may ruin your design.

- Start by practising simple designs, like a heart or a star, before trying more complicated ones. Breaking your design down into simple shapes can help you build up the image.

- When you've used all the polish up in your nail art pens, don't throw them away – refill them with your favourite colours.

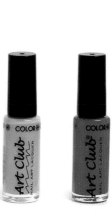

DOTTING TOOLS

The dotting tool comes in various sizes from tiny to large and double-ended; it can also be called different names such as a marbleizing tool or embossing tool. It is used to create dots or for swirling paint when marbleizing. It can also be used to pick up crystals, gems and rhinestones for placement.

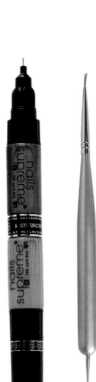

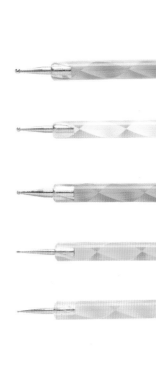

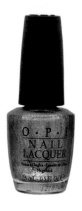
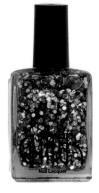
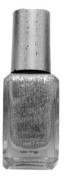
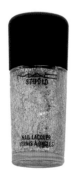
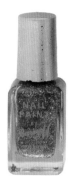

POLISHES & PAINTS

Nail polish is a product which, when applied, dries to a film-forming coat over the nail plate. There are many types of polish finishes to choose from, such as crème, matte, glitter, opalescent/iridescent, and metallic/chrome. Most of these finishes have been used in the nail art designs throughout the book.

Crème

This has a creamy finish that can be sheer or opaque.

Glitter

This has metallic glitter suspended in the polish and dries to a sparkly finish. It comes in a variety of colours, and shapes and sizes of particle. The particles make it hardwearing so it can be difficult to remove. Lots of remover, lint-free pads and patience is required. A quicker option is to invest in a peelable base coat. This can be applied before the glitter polish to ensure easy removal later on, with no damage to the natural nail.

Iridescent/Opalescent

Iridescent polish has reflective properties, which create a flash of colour when hit by light. Opalescent polish creates a pearlized finish.

Metallic/Chrome

These polishes create a highly polished finish, similar to metal.

Matte

This is a no-shine polish that dries to a matte finish. There are many matte nail polish products on the market with a variety of colours to choose from. Alternatively, you can purchase a mattifier or matte top coat to produce the effect and finish. Create contrasting texture by applying both matte and shiny finishes to your nail design.

Gel Polish

This is a popular product with clients and techs alike because of its shine and durability.

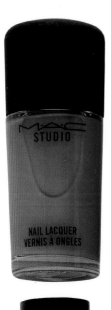
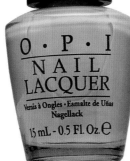
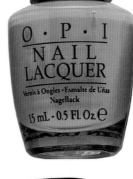
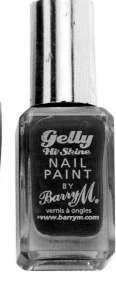
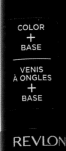
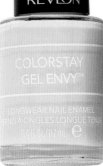
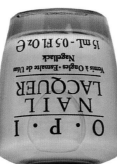
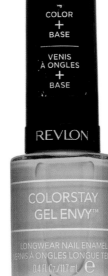
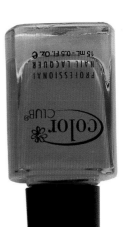

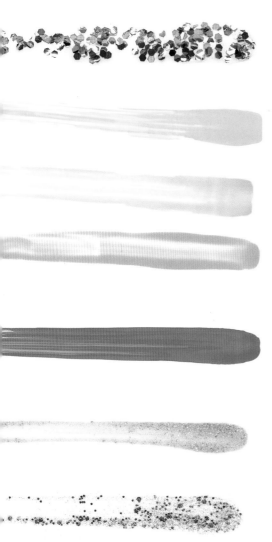

It is sometimes marketed as "the two-week manicure" as it lasts longer than regular polish without cracking, chipping or losing its shine. It is sometimes referred to as a soft gel as it is not as strong as the hard gels used to create nail extensions. It is applied in more or less the same way as regular polish, but it needs to be cured under a UV or LED lamp. As a consequence it needs to be removed professionally.

Acrylic Paint

Acrylic is a water-based paint that is commonly used in nail art. It is used for the artwork itself, not to paint the base nail colour. Available in a variety of colours, it can be easily mixed to create your own colour combinations. It's great for fine detail work as it has a thin consistency. It is relatively inexpensive to purchase and, as it is water based, if you make a mistake you can wipe it off fairly easily with water. It also dries quickly which is an advantage, and it's easy to remove with a nail wipe if you get it on the skin. Every nail artist has their own preferences on the medium they use for nail art. I suggest you try various types to find the one that suits your style and techniques.

APPLYING ALL-OVER COLOUR

When applying polish, do not overload your brush. You want to apply all coats in thin layers in order to get even colour coverage and so the layers dry quickly to prevent smudging. Working with less product on the brush also means you'll have more control. Take your time and rest your elbow on a surface to steady yourself, especially if you're using your non-dominant hand!

To paint an all-over base colour, paint the polish in three stripes down the nail. To avoid flooding the cuticle with polish, start a little towards the centre of the nail and push the paint towards the cuticle, making sure to leave a tiny gap. Then drag the polish towards the tip in a stripe in the centre of the nail. Paint another stripe down the left side and another on the right side, leaving a tiny gap all around the sidewalls.

If you do make a mistake, don't panic! You can always use a tidy-up brush dipped in polish remover to clean up and make the polish line around the cuticle picture perfect.

If you smudge a nail, you can easily fix it. Just dab your finger in polish remover and lightly tap the smudged area until it smoothes out the surface then finish with a top coat – as good as new!

PAINTING STRIPES

For perfect stripes, take your striping brush and dip it into your polish. Wipe off excess polish from the brush into the bottle so that the brush is coated evenly. Carefully lay the brush down onto the nail at the cuticle end and lightly drag the polish towards the tip. Clean your brush with nail polish remover each time you do a stripe as the build-up of polish on the brush will create uneven lines.

I find steadying your arm on a flat surface and holding your wrist lightly with your other hand helps if you're a little shaky.

TIPS FOR PAINTING THE DESIGNS

• Make sure each colour of your design is completely dry before applying another. If the first colour is still wet it can bleed into the next.

• Apply the first colour on all ten nails, and by the time you come back to the first nail to lay down another colour, it will be dry enough to apply.

• Always apply lighter colours first and darker colours and outlines on top of

these. Remember dark covers light but light may not cover dark!

• If you make a mistake, go with it and improvise – or stick gems over the areas you don't like!

• To steady your hand, use the little finger of your working hand and place it on the other little finger while painting. It's a little tricky at first but once you master it, it's sure worthwhile!

EMBELLISHMENTS

You can create so many different looks with the vast range of embellishments on the market. They can be used to add dimension and sparkle to your nail designs and are available in a range of shapes, colours and sizes. There are studs, pearls, gemstones, flatstones, crystals and tiny bullion beads as well as amazing stickers and transfers for super-quick and easy nail art. Shop around because the possibilities are endless!

Glitter

Glitter describes very small, flat, reflective particles that reflect light at different angles, causing the surface to sparkle and shimmer. Glitter is commonly manufactured from plastic. The glitter produced for the nail industry comes in small pots and is extra fine in texture, making it perfect for nail art as it is finer than craft glitter. It can be sprinkled over nail polish for a glitter gradient effect or used with top coat to form small beads to create individual designs and shapes. Extra top coat is usually required to seal the design to obtain a flat smooth surface. As well as the finer glitter, you can also use thicker craft glitters and/or glitter flakes to create textured effects.

Gemstones, Rhinestones and Crystals

Crystals and gemstones are commonly used in nail art. They are foil-backed, flat-back stones and can be purchased in many colours, shapes and sizes. They can also be referred to as rhinestones or diamantés. Crystals are generally of a better quality, Swarovski being the best-known example, and are therefore more expensive. You can also obtain acrylic gems which are less expensive, but the colours are not as bright and they can lose their lustre when used with a nail adhesive or top coat.

Studs

Studs are most commonly in gold and silver, but if you shop around you can usually obtain most colours – even neon and acid shades.

Pearls

Nail art pearls are made of plastic with a pearlized lustre coating, and are available in a variety of sizes, shapes and colours. You can purchase both flat-backed pearls and beads.

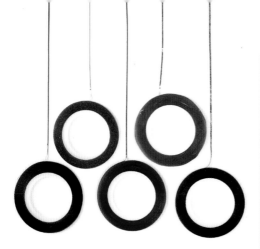

Striping Tape

Striping tape is a sticky-backed tape specially designed for nail art. It comes on tiny reels (see above) and in a variety of colours, thicknesses and textures, including glitter and metallic.

Stickers and Transfers

A great alternative to freehand nail art, as the design has already been created for you. Stickers usually come in an adhesive-backed sheet form, with a number of designs on the same sheet. You need to cut around the designs and then peel them off from the backing paper. Polish should be dry when applying stickers and then a top coat or finishing sealer applied to seal them.

Transfers also come in sheet form and need to be cut from the sheet. These are generally water based, and the backing paper needs to be dampened to release the transfer.

DECORATION TIPS

• When applying loose glitters with your top coat, be sure to wipe the brush clean before putting it back in the bottle.

• Use only good-quality gold bullion beads! Poor-quality types have a coating that comes off during the application of your top coat, spoiling your design!

• Where possible use good-quality crystal gems. Acrylic gems are less expensive but lose their lustre and shine when a top coat or nail adhesive is used. Swarovski crystals are best as they keep their sparkle.

• Flatstones are a by-product of sequins – the cut-out central bits – and are generally made from metallic foil. Be aware of the coloured ones, as the colour can run, thus spoiling your design. Use extra top coat to avoid dragging the flatstones.

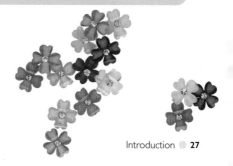

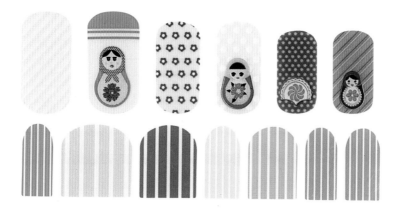

Once released, the transfer is placed onto the nail, smoothed over with a cotton bud and sealed with top coat or finishing sealer.

For both products, stork (embroidery) scissors are required to cut the designs from the sheet. A wooden manicure stick is useful to apply them to the nail, as both stickers and transfers can be fiddly. Tweezers can also be used.

Nail Art Wraps

These sticky-backed pre-designed coverings are usually applied with heat or pressure, or both, but always refer to manufacturer's instructions for application. They can be used to cover the whole nail, layered or cut into shapes and placed alongside other techniques to add an extra dimension to the design. Wraps are available in a variety of patterns, styles and finishes, are relatively easy to apply and can last one to two weeks. They require no drying time.

Nail Foils

Available in rolls or sheets in a variety of patterns and colours, foils are most commonly used for their highly metallic look. To use them, you will also need a foil adhesive.

The foil should be cut to shape, then the foil adhesive, which is usually white in colour, is applied to the nail and left to go clear. If there are any white patches remaining, the foil will not adhere. Once the adhesive is clear, the foil can be applied. The foil usually has the pattern or colour and shine on the top side and is dull underneath with no pattern. The dull side is applied to the adhesive, and the top of the foil is gently rubbed using a dry cotton bud to transfer the foil to the nail. A top coat or finishing sealer is then applied to seal and finish the design.

The adhesive generally comes in brush form but some suppliers do have foil adhesive in tubes or bottles with fine nozzles, allowing you to create detailed foil designs.

Gold and Silver Leaf

Gold and silver leaf – metal that has been hammered into extremely thin sheets – is often used for gilding. Real gold or silver can be used, but it can be expensive, and the less-expensive coloured metal leaf is the type usually used in nail art. The foil leaf can be applied to cover either the whole nail or only part of it. A top coat or nail adhesive is used to secure the leaf to the nail, and a top coat or finishing sealer must be applied to seal the design.

Nail Adhesive

These are fast-acting adhesives designed using chemical constituents – cyanoacrylates – developed for the nail industry. They are used to apply artificial nail tips to nails, generally to lengthen. Nail adhesives are also used to adhere nail gems, studs, pearls, and so on, to the nails for nail art.

Nail Enhancements and Press-ons

Nail enhancements are used to create length. An artificial nail tip creates the length while an overlay adds strength. The artificial tips are shaped nails made of plastic which are applied to the client's natural nails using nail adhesive and then overlaid with a choice of products that include acrylic, gel or wraps. The tips are generally applied to a third of the client's natural nail and the seam is blended before the overlay is applied. Because of natural nail growth, the enhancement will need to be maintained and rebalanced every two to four weeks.

Press-on nails or full-cover nails are also shaped nails made from plastic, but these are generally applied to the whole of the nail, hence the term "full-cover nail". Nail adhesive is also used to apply these, however they do not have an overlay applied and generally do not last as long – approximately one to two weeks. Press-on nails are usually the choice of session nail artists on photoshoots as they are quick and easy to apply, and can even be applied with double-sided tape for speedy removal after the shoot with no damage to the models' nails. They are available in a variety of shapes, lengths and styles and can be pre-prepared with nail art design and then applied when required.

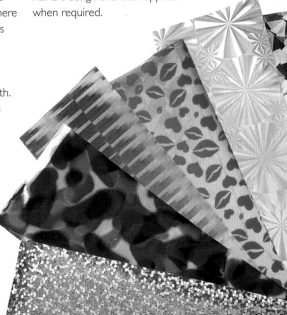

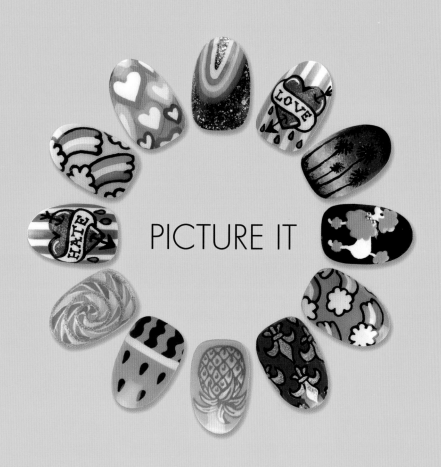

PICTURE IT

INTERGALACTIC RAINBOW

Create a manicure that's "out of this world" with a metallic glitter base and swirling rainbow stripes.

YOU WILL NEED:

grey metallic glitter polish, nail art pens or polish colours in red, orange, yellow, green and blue, striping brush (if not using pens), plus base coat and quick-dry top coat.

I After prepping and applying a base coat, apply two coats of grey metallic glitter to all 10 nails. If the glitter is quite chunky, it can be difficult to paint on top, so apply a quick-dry top coat after the two coats of glitter. This will give you a smoother base on which to draw the design. Leave to dry.

2 Using a red nail art pen or striping brush dipped in red nail polish, paint an S-shaped squiggly line from the cuticle to the tip. Paint different-shaped curved red outlines on the rest of the nails, some from tip to cuticle, others from side to side.

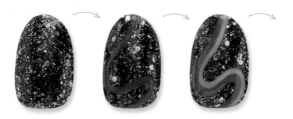

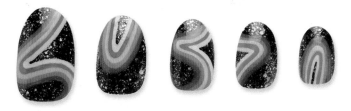

3 Using an orange nail art pen or a striping brush dipped in orange polish, paint a line following the shape of the red line but directly in front of it.

4 Repeat with the yellow polish, painting next to the orange line.

5 Paint a green line next to the yellow line.

6 Add a blue line, following the green line, to complete the rainbow effect.

7 When dry, seal with a top coat.

Option: You may prefer to paint the rainbow design on first and then fill in the sides with the glitter polish using a striping brush.

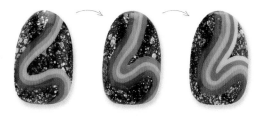

HEART TO HEART

Nails painted with a sweet heart motif make a pretty Valentine's treat.

YOU WILL NEED:

nail art pens or polish colours in pink, white, dark pink, yellow, light pastel green, dark blue and orange, fine detail brush (if not using pens), plus base coat and top coat.

1 After prepping and applying a base coat, apply two coats of pink polish to all 10 nails. Leave to dry.

2 Draw a heart on each nail using a white nail art pen or fine detail brush dipped in white polish.

3 Fill the whole nail up with hearts side by side and underneath and above the first heart.

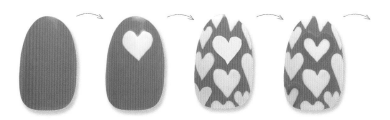

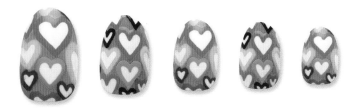

4   Using a dark pink nail art pen or fine detail brush dipped in dark pink polish, outline two of the hearts.

5   Outline two or three more hearts in yellow with a nail art pen or brush.

6   Outline other hearts in a light pastel green but make sure you leave enough hearts free to outline in two more colours!

7   Finish outlining the hearts in a dark blue and orange until you have outlined them all.

8   Leave to dry for a few minutes and then seal with a top coat.

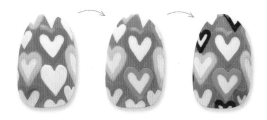

TATTOO HEARTS

*Use old-school sailor art
to send a message.*

YOU WILL NEED:

nail art pens or polish colours in white, pink, red glitter and black, striping brush and fine detail brush (if not using pens), plus base coat and top coat.

1   After prepping and applying a base coat, paint all 10 nails with two coats of white polish. Leave to dry.

2   Using a striping brush dipped in pink polish, paint vertical stripes on the nail from cuticle to tip.

3   When dry, paint a red glitter heart in the centre of each nail using a red glitter nail art pen or a fine detail brush dipped in red glitter polish. If your glitter is not very solid, draw the heart in red polish first and top with red glitter.

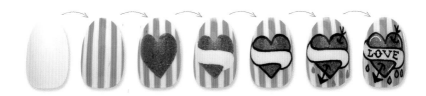

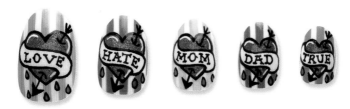

4　Using a white nail art pen or fine detail brush dipped in white polish, draw a banner shape across each of the hearts.

5　Outline the heart and banner with a black nail art pen or fine detail brush dipped in black polish.

6　Add a black arrow through the heart. Add three or four small red drips underneath the heart.

7　Using a black nail art pen or fine detail brush dipped in black polish, write LOVE inside the white banner in traditional tattoo-esque lettering.

8　Outline the drips in black and highlight the top and side of the heart with a curved line of white.

9　When dry, seal with a top coat.

For the Full Set: Vary the colour of the stripes and the words (try some tattoo themed words such as "HATE", "MOM", DAD" and "TRUE") on each nail, as illustrated above.

PALM SPRINGS

*Silhouettes of palm trees are set against
a vibrant island sunset.*

YOU WILL NEED:

*nail polish colours in black, purple, pink, yellow and green, aluminium foil, eyeshadow
sponge applicators, tissue, fine detail brush, plus base coat and top coat.*

1   Prep the nails and apply a base coat.

2   Pour a little black polish onto a piece of foil and dip a small eyeshadow
    sponge into the polish. Dab the excess onto a tissue, so the sponge is evenly
    coated. Starting at the tip of the nail, apply the colour about one-fifth down
    the length of the nail. Dab the sponge harder at the tip, going progressively
    lighter down the nail to achieve the faded effect. Leave enough space on the
    nail for four more colour fade stripes.

3   Repeat for all 10 nails and leave to dry. If you need a more solid covering of
    black at the tip, sponge a little more now and leave to dry again.

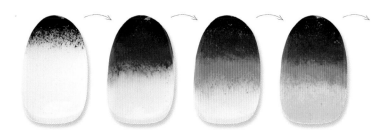

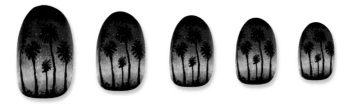

4   Repeat step 2 with the purple polish below the black. Sponge lightly over the fade of the black so the colours mix, creating a gradient colour effect.

5   Repeat with pink, yellow and green polishes to create further fades.

6   At the cuticle end, repeat the colour gradient with black. It's best to paint the black with a brush first, so you get a neat line, and then sponge the colour from there.

7   Using a fine detail brush dipped in black polish, draw five, slightly bent lines in varying sizes from the bottom black towards the tip, to represent the trunks of the palm trees.

8   Add bursts of black lines in different sizes from each end of the palm trunks to create the leaves. When dry, seal with a top coat.

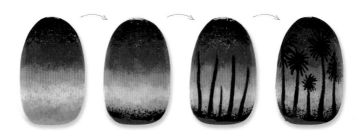

PINK POODLES

Get people "ooh la la"-ing over these pretty Parisian poodles!

YOU WILL NEED:

black and pink polish, nail art pens in pink, black and white, gold bullion beads, plus base coat and top coat.

1 Prep the nails and apply a base coat.

2 Paint alternate nails in two coats of pink and two coats of black. Leave to dry.

3 Using a white nail art pen, paint a small poodle head at the far left of each black nail, slightly below the tip. Start by drawing a circle and then elongate it to create a snout and draw a line below for the neck. (For the pink nails, follow the same steps using a black nail art pen.)

4 Draw the poodle's body by making a shape similar to a figure of eight on its side. The body should sit across the centre of the nail.

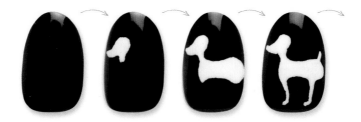

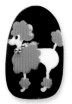

5 Draw two legs, with two dashes for the feet. Add a line for the poodle's tail.

6 Using a pink nail art pen, draw a cloud-like shape for the fur between the poodle's neck and front leg.

7 Add smaller pink cloud shapes to both legs just above the feet, and another cloud shape at the end of the tail. Draw another pink cloud shape of fur on top of the poodle's head, but make it slightly more curved to sit on the head.

8 Add a black dot to the poodle's face for an eye, and a pink dot at the tip of the snout for a nose. Add a white eye and nose for black poodles.

9 When dry, apply a top coat. While it is still wet, apply three gold bullion beads to the neck of the poodle for a collar. It's best to do this one nail at a time so the top coat remains wet. Finish with a second top coat to seal.

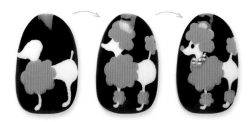

OVER THE RAINBOW

*Cast off cloudy days with these rainbows
in bursts of colour.*

YOU WILL NEED:

*lilac, yellow, green, peach and turquoise polishes, nail art pens or polish colours in pink,
turquoise, yellow, white and black, fine detail brush (if not using pens), plus base coat
and top coat.*

1   After prepping and applying a base coat, paint two coats of lilac polish
    over two nails (one on each hand). Repeat with yellow, green, orange and
    turquoise, so that you have different base colours on each hand.

2   Using a white nail art pen or a fine detail brush dipped in white polish, draw
    a little cloud shape on all 10 nails.

3   Add a rainbow shape (a thick, curved line) to the left-hand side of the cloud.

4   Continue painting cloud and rainbow shapes until you have covered the nail,
    making sure to leave enough space between each one.

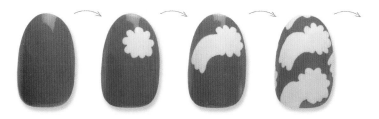

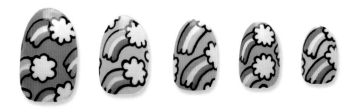

5   Using a pink nail art pen or fine detail brush dipped in pink, add a stripe to the top curve of the rainbow shapes. You will want the pink to cover one-third of the white.

6   Leave the same width of white and then add a stripe of turquoise to the lower curve of the rainbow, again the same thickness as the pink stripe.

7   Add yellow stripes to some clouds so that you have some pink/white/turquoise and some yellow/white/turquoise rainbow combinations.

8   Outline the cloud and rainbow with a black nail art pen or fine detail brush dipped in black polish.

9   When dry, seal with a top coat.

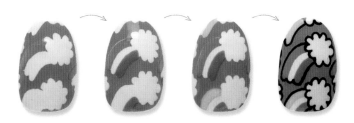

FLEUR-DE-LIS

Give your nails their very own coat of arms with these gold heraldic motifs.

YOU WILL NEED:

nail art pens or polish colours in royal blue, gold, black and gold glitter, fine detail brush (if not using pens), plus base coat and top coat.

1 After prepping and applying a base coat, paint all 10 nails with two coats of royal blue. Leave to dry.

2 Using a gold nail art pen or fine detail brush dipped in gold polish, draw a pointed "leaf" shape at the tip of the nail.

3 Either side of the first "leaf" shape, paint a curved sideways crescent shape in gold and extend the "body" of the fleur-de-lis slightly downwards.

4 Draw a gold line down from the "body" of the fleur-de-lis.

5 Paint two smaller curved crescent shapes the opposite way around to the first crescent shapes, coming from either side of the line.

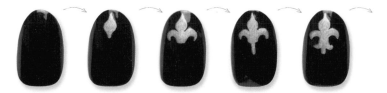

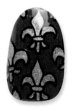

6 Continuing with the gold, repeat the steps to create another fleur-de-lis below the first. You probably won't be able to fit in another complete shape, so keep them the same size but paint part of one in the space remaining.

7 Paint two more fleur-de-lis shapes at the side of each nail, in the spaces between the first two. Paint the bottom of a fleur-de-lis in the spaces left at the tip, so you have an overall fleur-de-lis print effect.

8 Using a black nail art pen or fine detail brush dipped in black polish, outline the bottom half of the fleur-de-lis, so that you have three separate petals coming from an outlined "toggle" shape.

9 Outline the top "leaf" shape and crescent-shaped petals of the fleur-de-lis in black.

10 Add gold glitter detailing to the gold motifs. Seal with a top coat.

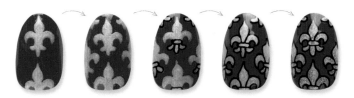

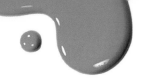

PASTEL PINEAPPLES

Subtly shaded pineapples give a burst of fruity flavour to your fingertips!

YOU WILL NEED:

nail art pens or polish colours in pastel pink, white, yellow, turquoise and pastel blue, fine detail brush (if not using pens), plus base coat and top coat.

1 Prep all 10 nails, apply a base coat and then paint two coats of pastel pink polish. Leave to dry.

2 At the bottom of each nail, paint a circle with a white nail art pen or fine detail brush dipped in white polish.

3 Paint five white pineapple leaf shapes coming out of the top of the circle.

4 Using a yellow nail art pen or fine detail brush dipped in yellow polish, add shadow detail to the pineapple leaves and a crescent moon shape to the body of the pineapple.

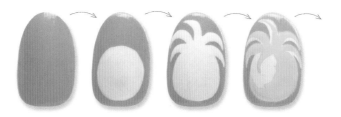

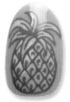

5 Using a turquoise nail art pen or fine detail brush dipped in turquoise polish, outline the leaves and the body of the pineapple.

6 With the same turquoise colour, paint a criss-cross pattern inside the body of the pineapple and lines in the centre of each leaf.

7 Using a pastel blue nail art pen or fine detail brush dipped in pastel blue polish, paint shadow detailing in half of the diamond shapes in the grid on the body of the pineapple.

8 Using the turquoise nail art pen or polish, paint a dash in each diamond shape of the grid on the body of the pineapple.

9 When all 10 nails are complete and dry, seal with a top coat.

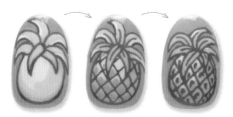

FRUIT COCKTAIL

Go tropical with this fruity manicure. Try a different fruit on each nail for a fun fruit cocktail!

YOU WILL NEED:

nail art pens or polish colours in neon coral, lime green, white, dark green, black, yellow and brown, striping brush, fine detail brush (if not using pens), dotting tool, plus base coat and top coat.

Watermelons

1   Prep and apply a base coat, then paint the nails in neon coral. Leave to dry.

2   Paint one-third of the nail at the tip or cuticle end using a striping brush dipped in lime green polish. Leave to dry. Between the green and the neon coral, paint a thick white line using a striping brush with polish.

3   Using a dark green nail art pen or fine detail brush dipped in dark green polish, paint squiggly vertical stripes over the lime green. With a dotting tool and black polish, add three dots in a line, then two dots in a line, on the coral.

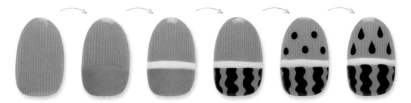

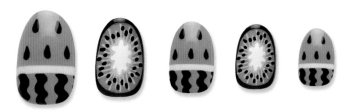

4 Using a black nail art pen or fine detail brush dipped in black, elongate the dots so they look like watermelon seeds! When dry, apply a top coat.

Kiwi Fruit

1 After prepping and applying a base coat, paint the nails with lime green polish.

2 Using a white nail art pen or fine detail brush dipped in white polish, paint a large "flower" shape, or core, in the centre of the nail. Leave to dry, then paint thin lines, uneven in length, radiating out from the "flower".

3 With a nail art pen or fine detail brush, outline the "flower" in yellow.

4 Using a dotting tool and black polish, make small black dots to represent seeds. Using a striping or fine detail brush and brown polish, draw a line around the outside to create the skin. Make the line slightly thicker at the top and bottom of the nail for a 3D effect. When dry, apply a top coat.

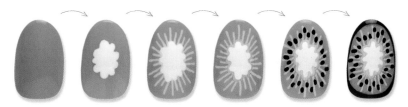

CANDY SWIRL

Get sweet-shop style with painted pinwheel lollipops.

YOU WILL NEED:

nail art pens or polish colours in white, silver glitter, neon pink, green, blue and orange, fine detail brush (if not using pens), plus base coat and top coat.

1   After prepping and applying a base coat, paint two coats of white polish on all 10 nails.

2   Using a silver glitter nail art pen or fine detail brush dipped in silver glitter polish, paint a swirl from the centre of the nail all the way out to the edge. Paint a silver outline all the way around the nail.

3   Using a neon pink nail art pen or fine detail brush dipped in neon pink polish, paint a small crescent-shaped section at the beginning of the swirl in the centre of the nail.

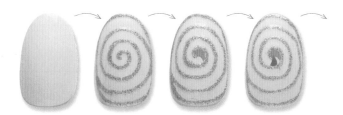

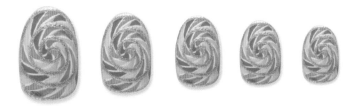

4   Leave a small line of white and paint another section using a green nail art pen or fine detail brush dipped in green polish. Each colour section needs to curve around the swirl in a crescent shape.

5   Paint blue and orange crescent sections, leaving small lines of white between each colour.

6   Repeat with yellow, leaving a small line of white in between.

7   Continue painting crescent shapes, ever-increasing in size and changing in colour. You can alternate colours if you like!

8   Repeat the whole way around the swirl until you have filled the entire nail.

9   When dry, seal with a top coat.

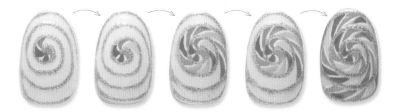

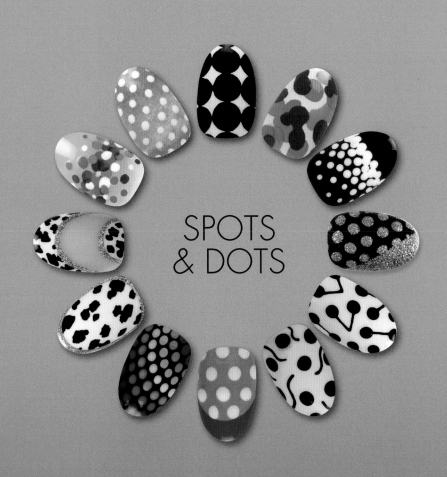

SPOTS
& DOTS

'60S MONOCHROME SPOTS

Create eye-catching Op Art at your fingertips with this "spot-on" design.

YOU WILL NEED:

nail art pens or polish colours in white and black, fine detail brush (if not using pens), plus base coat and top coat.

1 After prepping the nails and applying a base coat, apply two coats of white polish to all 10 nails.

2 Draw a black circle in the centre of each nail with a black nail art pen or fine detail brush dipped in black polish.

3 Fill in the circle with black.

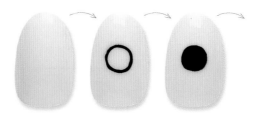

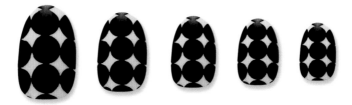

4   Paint a circle either side of the centre circle, so that each is touching in a row across the nail.

5   Paint another three circles directly above the first row of circles, making sure they are all touching.

6   Paint another three circles below the first row of circles.

7   Paint rows of half-circles top and bottom so the whole nail is covered with the design.

8   When all the nails are completed and the polish is dry, apply a top coat.

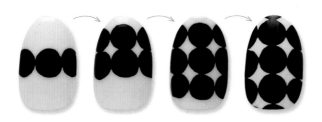

LAVA LAMP

Psychedelic bubbles of colour
create a fun retro look.

YOU WILL NEED:

cream polish, nail art pens or polish colours in green, lilac, red and blue, fine detail brush (if not using pens), plus base coat and top coat.

1   After prepping the nails and applying a base coat, paint two coats of cream polish on all 10 nails.

2   Using a green nail art pen or fine detail brush dipped in green polish, paint irregular circle shapes over the nail. Try painting a circle and then a larger circle above or below it to give you a figure-of-eight shape. Leave to dry.

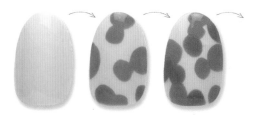

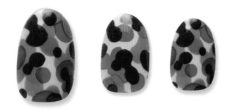

3 Repeat using a lilac nail art pen or fine detail brush dipped in lilac polish, painting irregular circle shapes in the cream spaces and also overlapping some of the lilac circles with the green.

4 Repeat with a red nail art pen or polish, again overlapping colours.

5 Repeat with a blue nail art pen or polish, layering over the other colours.

6 When dry, seal with a top coat.

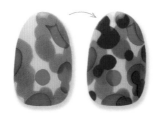

DOTTY GRADIENT DESIGN

Go dotty with this super-simple navy-and-white gradient.

YOU WILL NEED:

nail polish colours in dark blue and white, dotting tool, plus base coat and top coat.

1   After prepping the nails and applying a base coat, apply two coats of dark blue polish to all 10 nails.

2   Using a dotting tool dipped in white polish, paint a row of dots across the nail, a little way down from the tip.

3   Add another two rows of dots directly below the first row of dots, but placing the dots in the spaces between the first row of dots to create a dotty zig-zag.

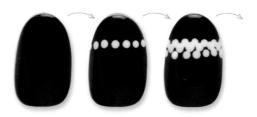

4   Keep adding more dots below the existing rows of dots, but this time position them more randomly and not so close together.

5   Continue adding dots down the nail, placing them further apart from each other and also making them slightly smaller to create a gradient of dots.

6   When dry, seal with a top coat.

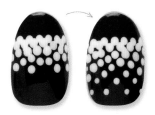

TOP TIP

• You can buy dotting tools in all different sizes. Try using the biggest size first, working in progressively smaller sizes to create the gradient effect.

GLITTER POLKA DOTS

Bronze and gold glitter polishes give a textured 3D effect to this asymmetrical dot design.

YOU WILL NEED:

nail polish colours in black, gold glitter and bronze glitter, striping brush, dotting tool, plus base coat and top coat.

1   After prepping the nails and applying a base coat, apply two coats of black nail polish to all 10 nails.

2   Using a striping brush dipped in gold glitter polish, paint a diagonal section of gold at the right-hand tip of the nail.

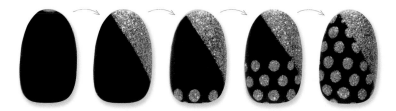

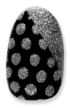

3 Using a dotting tool dipped in a bronze glitter polish, apply a row of dots at the cuticle end of the nail.

4 Keep adding bronze glitter dots in rows above the first line of dots, all the way up to the diagonal gold glitter tip.

5 When dry, seal with a top coat.

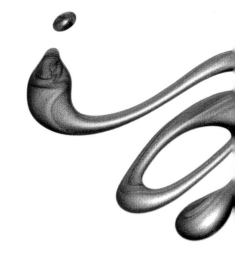

TOP TIPS

• *For a textured glitter effect, don't apply a top coat.*

• *To keep your dots even and consistent, wipe clean the dotting tool between dot placement.*

'80S ATOMS

You'll be in your element creating this atomic motif for a retro-inspired design.

YOU WILL NEED:

nail art pens or polish colours in bright yellow, white and black, dotting tool and fine detail brush (if not using pens), plus base coat and top coat.

Yellow Design

1   After prepping the nails and applying a base coat, apply two coats of bright yellow polish to five alternating nails. (The other five nails are painted white, as detailed opposite.)

2   Using a black nail art pen or dotting tool dipped in black polish, paint a circle.

3   Paint more black circles in a random pattern, making sure they are all the same size and that you leave some space between them to paint the lines.

4   Using a black nail art pen or fine detail brush dipped in black polish, paint a squiggly line between two of the circles. Add a few more squiggles.

5   When dry, seal with a top coat.

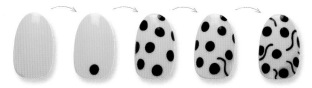

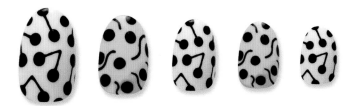

White Design

1 Paint the other five nails with two coats of white polish over the base coat.

2 Using a black nail art pen or dotting tool dipped in black polish, paint a circle on the left side of the nail in the centre.

3 Paint another circle, the same size as the first circle, diagonally below it and to the right.

4 Join the two circles together with a black V-shaped line, so that they resemble two atoms joined together.

5 Above the "atoms" paint two more black circles and join them together with a straight line.

6 Keep painting the same design of "atoms" until you have an all-over pattern.

7 When dry, seal with a top coat.

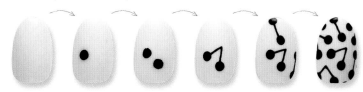

DOTTY FRENCH MANICURE

A bold French-tip colour makes these spotted nails really pop!

YOU WILL NEED:

nail polish colours in light denim blue, bright blue and off-white, striping brush, dotting tool, plus base coat and top coat.

1 After prepping the nails and applying a base coat, paint two coats of light denim blue polish on all 10 nails.

2 Using a striping brush dipped in bright blue polish, paint a French tip on each nail.

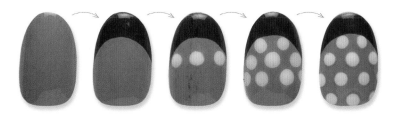

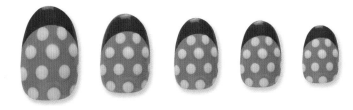

3 Using a dotting tool dipped in off-white polish, paint three spots across the nail, slightly below the French tip.

4 Add another row of spots below the first, then add two spots directly on the line where the French tip meets the lighter blue. Add rows of spots all the way down the nail.

5 When dry, seal with a top coat.

TOP TIP

• *To paint perfect French tips, use dots as a guide. First paint a dot in the centre of the nail where you want the highest arch of the tip to be, then paint a dot on either side of the central dot, slightly lower down, to create a guide for an even curve. Fill in the tip using a striping brush.*

RAINBOW DOTS

Add a spectrum of rainbow colours to a solid black background for an eye-catching display.

YOU WILL NEED:

nail art pens or polish colours in black, dark blue, light blue, light green, yellow, orange, red and purple, dotting tool (if not using pens), plus base coat and top coat.

1   After prepping the nails and applying a base coat, paint all 10 nails with two coats of black polish.

2   Using a dark blue nail art pen or dotting tool dipped in dark blue nail polish, paint a curved line of spots running diagonally in the bottom right-hand corner of the nail.

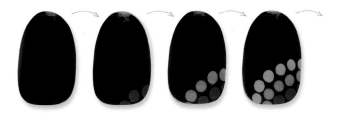

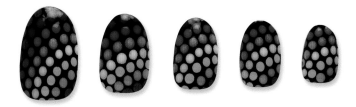

3   Using a light blue nail art pen or dotting tool dipped in light blue polish, paint spots above the dark blue line, following the curved diagonal.

4   Repeat with light green spots just above the light blue, followed by yellow, orange and red spots.

5   Finish with a line of purple spots above the red.

6   When all the nails are complete and the spots are dry, seal with a top coat.

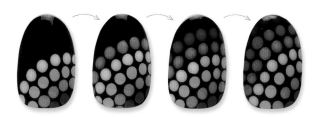

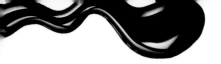

DALMATIAN SPOTS

Gold glitter adds a touch of sparkle to these canine-inspired creations, while nude negative space keeps it chic and modern.

YOU WILL NEED:

nail art pens or polish colours in white, black, gold glitter, nude, fine detail brush and striping brush (if not using pens), plus base coat and top coat.

All-over Spots

1. After prepping the nails and applying a base coat, paint four feature nails with two coats of white polish. (The other six nails are painted nude, as detailed opposite.)

2. Using a black nail art pen or fine detail brush dipped in black polish, paint an irregular-shaped "dalmatian" spot.

3. Continue painting random "dalmatian" spots – big and small, some close together, some touching, some further apart – around the entire nail.

4. Using a fine detail brush dipped in gold glitter polish, paint a thin outline around the nail. When dry, seal with a top coat.

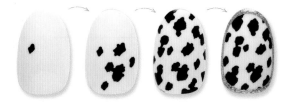

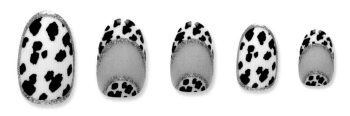

Spotty Tips

1   Paint the other six nails with two coats of nude polish over the base coat.

2   Using a white nail art pen or striping brush dipped in white polish, paint a French tip on the nude nails.

3   Paint a white half moon on the nails.

4   Using a black nail art pen or fine detail brush dipped in black polish, paint "dalmatian" spots on the half moon and French tip.

5   Using a striping brush or fine detail brush dipped in gold glitter polish, paint a line underneath the French tip and above the half moon. Leave to dry and seal with a top coat.

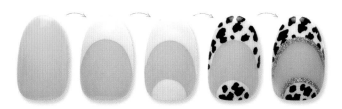

SEE-THROUGH SPOTS

Bubbles of colour cleverly combine with a clear base to create this spotty showstopper.

YOU WILL NEED:

nail polish colours in lime green, dark green, pink, purple, orange, blue and cream, striping brush, dotting tool, plus base coat and top coat.

1 After prepping the nails and applying a base coat, paint half of each nail with a striping brush dipped in lime green polish, leaving the rest the natural nail base.

2 Using a dotting tool dipped in dark green polish, paint random dots in different sizes above, below and on the dividing line of lime green. Make the dots smaller the further away they are from the dividing lime green line.

3 Repeat with pink dots, clustering them on and around the dividing line.

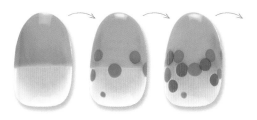

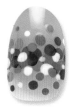

4 Repeat, adding dots in purple and orange.

5 Repeat with blue dots until the line between the lime green polish and the clear base coat is covered and you have dots spreading out in a slight gradient effect.

6 On top of the coloured cluster of dots, add some cream-coloured dots in different sizes, spreading them out like a gradient effect.

7 When the dots are dry, seal with a top coat.

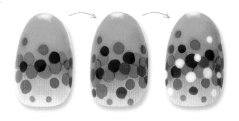

TOP TIP

• *If you are creating this effect on false nails, choose clear plastic tips to get the negative-space effect.*

RAINBOW GRADIENT POLKA DOTS

Colour fades make a pretty background for this twist on a classic polka-dot design.

YOU WILL NEED:

nail polish colours in pink, blue, green, yellow, orange and white, eyeshadow sponge applicators, tissue, dotting tool or nail art pen in white, aluminium foil, plus base coat and top coat.

1   Prep the nails and apply a base coat.

2   Pour a little pink polish onto a piece of foil and dip a small makeup sponge into the polish. Dab the excess onto a tissue so the sponge is evenly coated. Sponge the pink lightly onto the tip of the nail. Dab the sponge harder at the tip to apply more polish, and more lightly as you move down the nail to achieve the faded effect. Make sure you leave enough space on the nail for four more colour fade stripes.

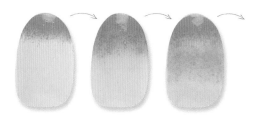

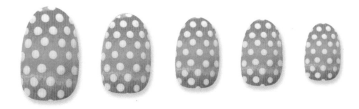

3   Repeat with blue polish directly under the pink, making sure to sponge a little into the pink to create a soft fade.

4   Repeat with green, yellow and orange colours.

5   Using a white nail art pen or a dotting tool dipped in white polish, make polka dots in horizontal rows across the rainbow fade. The dots should be evenly spaced and each row of dots should be offset so the dots do not line up vertically.

6   Continue adding rows of polka dots until the whole nail is covered.

7   When dry, seal with a top coat.

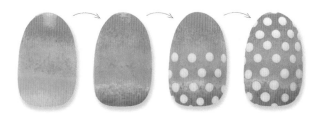

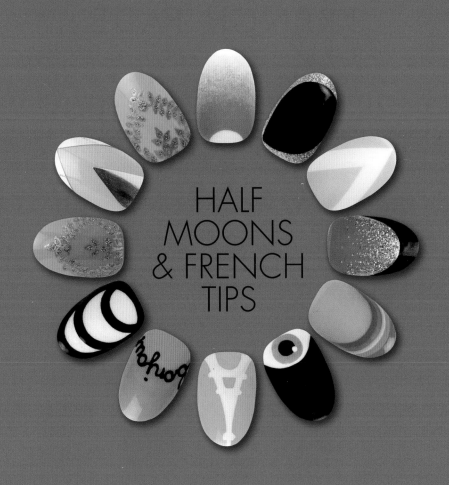

HALF
MOONS
& FRENCH
TIPS

FRENCH FADE

Update your look with this modern twist on the classic pink-and-white French tip and half moon manicure.

YOU WILL NEED:

nail polish colours in nude, cream and white, eyeshadow sponge applicators, aluminium foil, tissue, striping brush, plus base coat and top coat.

1   Prep the nails and apply a base coat. Apply two coats of nude polish on all 10 nails. Leave to dry.

2   Pour a little cream polish onto a piece of foil and dip an eyeshadow sponge applicator into the polish. Dab the excess onto a tissue so the sponge is evenly coated. Very lightly sponge the cream colour onto the top half of the nail, so that it's partially covered with some of the nude still showing through.

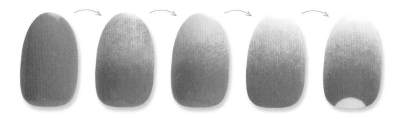

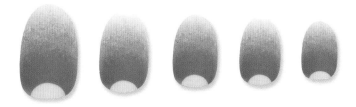

3   Dab the tip of the nail with more cream colour, so that the top half is filled in, while the bottom half is slightly transparent.

4   Dip a clean sponge into white polish, remove the excess as before, and apply to the tip of the nail, following the curve of the nail tip.

5   With a striping brush dipped in white polish, draw and fill in a half moon shape at the base of the nail.

6   When dry, seal with a top coat.

TOP TIPS

• *You can use a small makeup sponge to create gradient effects but I prefer an eyeshadow sponge applicator as it gives more control and means less mess over the cuticle and surrounding skin.*

• *Always dab off excess polish from the sponge to get a light level of coverage you can build on.*

• *Make sure the colour is dry before dabbing on more - if still wet, the sponge will remove colour rather than add it .*

BLACK & GOLD

You can't beat classic black and gold for a hint of sultry midnight glamour.

YOU WILL NEED:

nail polish colours in gold glitter and black, striping brush, plus base coat and matte top coat.

1 After prepping the nails and applying a base coat, apply two coats of gold glitter to all 10 nails. Leave to dry.

2 Using a striping brush, paint a black curved line from the lower left corner to the upper right of each nail except the ring fingers (see opposite), leaving a 2 mm (1/16 inch) gap.

3 Paint another curved line along the bottom to create a "lemon" shape, again leaving a 2 mm (1/16 inch) gap of gold.

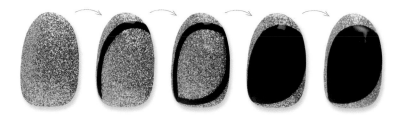

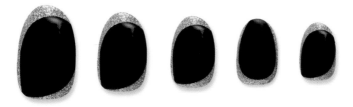

4 Fill in the "lemon" shape with black polish.

5 Paint a matte top coat over the black, leaving the gold glitter shiny.

Ring Fingers

1 After applying two coats of gold glitter polish, paint black polish over the gold using the brush in the polish bottle. Leave a 2 mm (¹⁄₁₆ inch) gap above the cuticle and start by painting a stripe of black polish towards the tip.

2 Curve the brush around and paint the sides, making sure to leave the gap of gold at the cuticle and side walls of the nail.

3 Apply a matte top coat to the black, leaving the gold shiny.

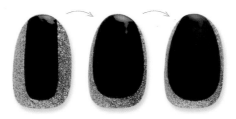

CHEVRON BLEU

A matte top coat gives this clean, geometric design a modern finish.

YOU WILL NEED:

nail polish colours in mint blue and white, striping brush, plus base coat and matte top coat.

1 After prepping nails and applying a base coat, paint all 10 nails with two coats of mint blue polish. Leave to dry.

2 Using a striping brush dipped in white polish, make a diagonal line from the right-hand side of the base to the left side of the tip of each nail.

3 Make another white diagonal line from the left-hand side of the base of the nail to the right-hand side of the tip, to create a triangle shape.

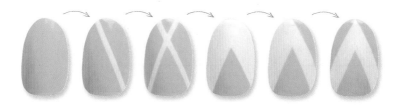

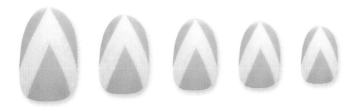

4   Fill in the tip area within the crossing lines with white polish, leaving a blue triangle at the cuticle end of the nail.

5   Paint a diagonal tip using a striping brush dipped in mint blue polish at the right-hand side of the nail, ending in the centre of the tip.

6   Paint another mint blue tip line on the left-hand side, meeting the other blue line in the centre of the tip to leave a white chevron in the centre of the nail.

7   When dry, seal with a matte top coat.

TOP TIP

• *To ensure your chevrons are all the same size and centred, first place two white dots at the cuticle end to mark the width of the base of the triangle. Then place another dot where you want the point of the triangle to be. Do this for all nails and then connect the dots with lines as for steps 2 and 3.*

GLITTER GRADIENT

The turquoise colour and silver glitter give a stunning, jewel-like effect to the nails.

YOU WILL NEED:

nail polish colours in turquoise, black, silver and silver glitter, striping brush, fine detail brush, plus base coat and top coat.

1   After prepping the nails and applying a base coat, paint all 10 nails with two coats of turquoise nail polish. Leave to dry.

2   Add a curved French tip to each nail using a striping brush dipped in black polish.

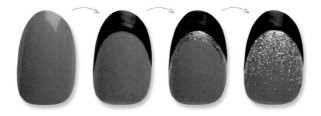

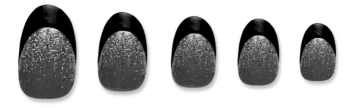

3 Underneath the black French tip, add a line of silver polish using the striping brush dipped in silver polish.

4 Using a fine detail brush, brush on silver glitter polish, starting from the silver line in a gradient effect towards the cuticle.

5 When all 10 nails are complete and the glitter is dry, seal with a top coat.

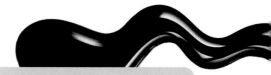

TOP TIP

• *If you find French tips difficult, try using paper reinforcement rings for a perfect, clean curve every time! Make sure to place them on fully dried polish and position the curve of the reinforcer below the tip line. Paint your tip and remove the reinforcer immediately before the polish dries.*

RAINBOW TIPS

*Top off your nails with this
sunny-day rainbow.*

YOU WILL NEED:

nail polish colours in nude, blue, green, yellow, orange and red, striping brush, plus base coat and top coat.

1   After prepping the nails and applying a base coat, paint all 10 nails with two coats of nude polish. Leave to dry.

2   Using a striping brush dipped in blue polish, paint a curved line about one-quarter of the way down the nail from the tip.

3   Above this, paint a green line directly above the blue.

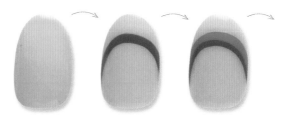

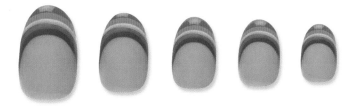

4 Paint a yellow curved line directly above the green.

5 Paint an orange line directly above the yellow.

6 Finish the rainbow tip with a red line above the orange, so the red line
is sitting right at the tip.

7 When dry, seal with a top coat.

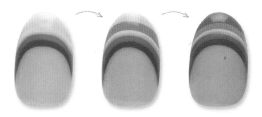

EYE OF THE MOON

*Ward off evil spirits with this
eye-catching half moon design!*

YOU WILL NEED:

nail polish colours in black, white and blue, striping brush, fine detail brush and dotting tool, plus base coat and top coat.

1   After prepping the nails and applying a base coat, paint all 10 nails with two coats of black polish. Leave to dry.

2   Paint a white half moon on each nail using a striping brush dipped in white polish.

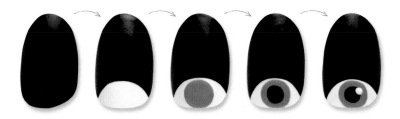

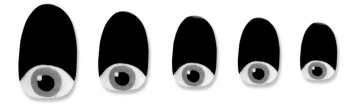

3 Using a fine detail brush dipped in blue polish, paint a circle in the centre of the white half moon.

4 Using a dotting tool dipped in black polish, paint a smaller black circle inside the blue circle.

5 Add a white dot where the blue and black circles meet, to the top right of the black circle, with the dotting tool.

6 When dry, seal with a top coat.

TOP TIP

• *If you find half moons difficult to do, try using paper reinforcement rings. Instead of black, start with a white base and place a reinforcement ring at the cuticle end of the nail to create the half-circle. Paint the rest of the nail black, then remove the ring carefully before the polish dries.*

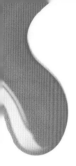

A VERY FRENCH MANICURE

Say "bonjour" with this pretty pink-and-turquoise French manicure.

YOU WILL NEED:

nail polish colours in pink, turquoise and black, striping brush, fine detail brush, black nail art pen, plus base coat and top coat.

1   After prepping the nails and applying a base coat, paint all 10 nails with two coats of pink polish. Leave to dry.

2   Using a striping brush dipped in turquoise polish, paint a line to form a half moon and then fill in the nail from the top of the half moon to the tip, so you're left with a pink half moon.

TOP TIP

• *Practise writing words in script lettering on paper beforehand.*

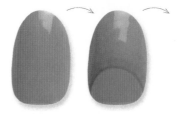

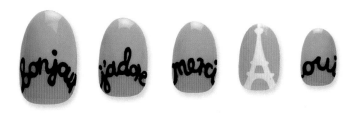

3   Using a black nail art pen or fine detail brush dipped in black polish, start writing "bonjour" in curly writing at the left-hand side of the half moon, where the turquoise and pink meet.

4   Continue spelling out "bonjour" along the line of the half moon, making sure that you go right across to the other side of the nail.

5   When dry, seal with a top coat.

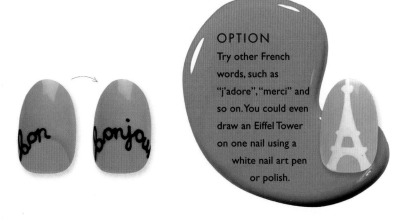

OPTION

Try other French words, such as "j'adore", "merci" and so on. You could even draw an Eiffel Tower on one nail using a white nail art pen or polish.

'60S OP-ART OUTLINE

Make a graphic statement with this bold black-and-white outlined design.

YOU WILL NEED:

nail polish colours in white and black, striping brush, plus base coat and top coat.

I After prepping the nails and applying a base coat, paint all 10 nails with two coats of white polish. Leave to dry.

2 Using a striping brush dipped in black polish, paint an outline all the way around the nail.

3 Paint a half-moon line in black.

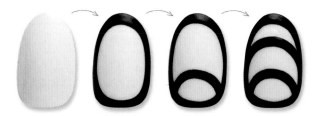

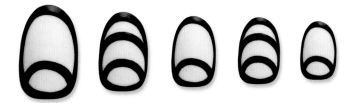

4   Paint a curved line about one-quarter of the way down from the tip to create an outlined French tip.

5   When dry, seal with a top coat.

For the Full Set: Leave some of the nails with just outlined half moons and some with outlined French tips!

TOP TIP

• *Don't panic if you make a mistake with the black. You can always make corrections by using a brush dipped in nail polish remover to clean up and neaten lines or by using white polish to hide any mistakes. The top coat will smooth out any polish build-up.*

INDIAN SUMMER

Slip into summer with this exotic nail design inspired by intricate Indian sari patterns.

YOU WILL NEED:

nail art pens or polish colours in bright blue, coral, gold and gold glitter, striping brush and fine detail brush (if not using pens), plus base coat and top coat.

1 After prepping the nails and applying a base coat, paint two coats of bright blue nail polish to all 10 nails. Leave to dry.

2 Paint a chevron French tip using a coral nail art pen or striping brush dipped in coral polish.

3 Using a gold nail art pen or a fine detail brush dipped in gold polish, paint a small pointed "leaf" shape over the point where the coral and blue meet. Add a gold leaf both sides of this.

4 Paint a gold outlined circle, joining the last two "leaves" together, then from either side of the circle, draw two curved lines and a "leaf" shape at the end of both lines.

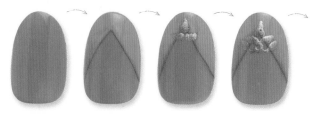

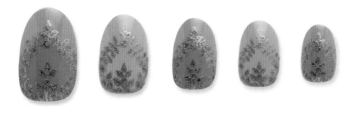

5 Following the diagonal line of the coral polish, paint a line of two "leaf" shapes side by side on the right-hand side of the nail.

6 Repeat on the left-hand side of the nail.

7 At the cuticle end of the nail, paint a pointed leaf shape with two more leaves either side, a circle underneath this, and then a line down to the cuticle. Coming from either side of this line, draw two more "leaves".

8 Right at the cuticle line, paint leaves all along, outlining the whole base of the nail until you reach each side of the chevron tip.

9 Add gold glitter detailing to the gold "leaves".

10 When dry, seal with a top coat.

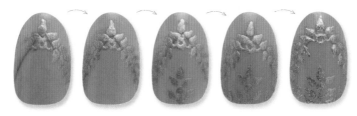

V.I.T. (VERY IMPORTANT TIPS!)

Get VIP status with these gold foil chevron nails.

YOU WILL NEED:

nail polish in nude, gold nail art foil stickers, plus base coat and top coat.

1   After prepping the nails and applying a base coat, paint all 10 nails with two coats of nude polish. Leave to dry.

2   Cut out 10 triangle shapes with a slightly curved bottom (so that they fit into the line of the cuticle) from gold nail art foil stickers. Apply the triangles to each nail at the cuticle end – the foil has a sticky back so should just stick to the nail. You can push down gently using a cotton bud (Q-tip) to smooth them out, but make sure your nude colour is completely dry.

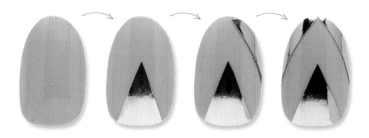

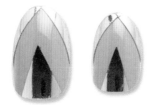

3 Cut out a thin strip of gold foil and place on the right-hand side of the nail tip in a diagonal towards the centre of the tip. Press down and smooth out. Then file the tip in a downwards motion to remove the excess foil. The foil should now be flush at the tip.

4 Repeat, applying a gold strip diagonally at the left-hand side to meet the right-hand strip in the centre of the tip.

5 Seal with a top coat.

TOP TIP

• Use stork (embroidery) scissors to cut the gold foil and use a wooden stick or tweezers to hold the foil in position for placement.

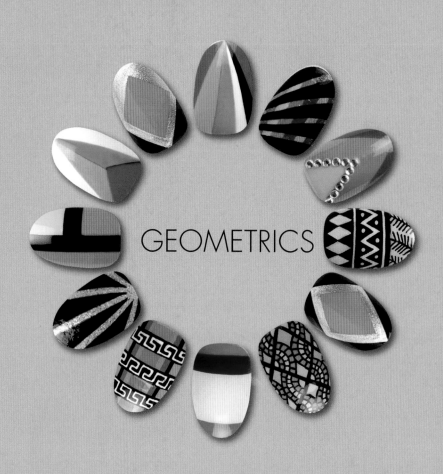

GEOMETRICS

NEON PRISM

These 3D geometrics can be painted in any colour combination you like but neon has mega-watt impact.

YOU WILL NEED:

nail polish colours in white, neon purple, neon orange, black and neon green, striping brush, plus base coat and top coat.

1 Prep nails and apply a base coat, then paint two coats of white polish on all 10 nails. Leave to dry.

2 Using a striping brush dipped in neon purple polish, draw a line from the centre of the tip of the nail to just above the right-hand corner of the cuticle at the bottom. Fill in the section with the purple colour.

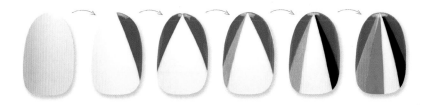

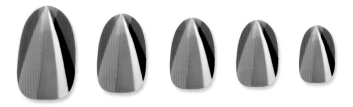

3 Using the same purple colour, repeat from the centre of the tip to just above the left-hand corner of the cuticle at the bottom and fill in again. You should be left with a triangle of white in the centre of the nail.

4 You will now divide the white triangle into four equal strips of colour. To do this, use a striping brush dipped in neon orange polish to paint a line next to the purple line and one-quarter of the way into the triangle. Fill in with colour.

5 Do the same on the opposite side with a striping brush dipped in black polish.

6 Using a striping brush dipped in neon green polish, draw a dividing line through the middle of the remaining white triangle. Fill in with colour.

7 When dry, seal with a top coat.

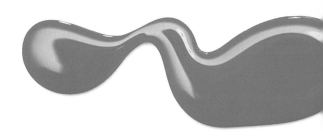

STROBE LIGHTS

Get disco fever with these flashing effects — or simply stop at step 5 for a multicolour striped design.

YOU WILL NEED:

nail polish colours in white, neon green, neon yellow, neon orange, red, blue, pink and black, striping brush, gemstone-effect overcoat, plus top coat..

1 Paint all 10 nails with two thin coats of white polish. This step is not essential, but the neon colours really pop on a white base. Leave to dry.

2 Using a striping brush dipped in neon green polish, paint a stripe down each nail. You can vary the placement of the green stripe for each nail but keep them roughly the same width. The good thing about this technique is that you don't have to be too precise with your stripes, as the black sections will mostly cover them.

3 Using a striping brush dipped in neon yellow polish, paint a stripe directly next to the neon green stripe, keeping the stripes roughly the same thickness.

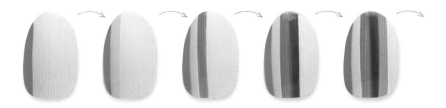

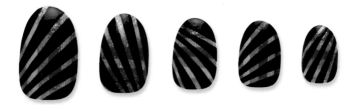

4   Repeat to create neon orange, red, neon pink, blue and purple stripes.

5   When dry, apply gemstone-effect overcoat.

6   When the overcoat is dry, dip a striping brush in black polish and paint a diagonal stripe across the colourful stripes at one top corner.

7   Paint a fan-shaped black strip next to the one you have just painted, leaving a thin gap of the colourful stripes in-between.

8   Paint four black diagonal stripes in fan shapes radiating from the side, leaving colourful gaps between them. Finish with a final black fan at the cuticle end.

9   When dry, seal with a top coat.

For the Full Set: Vary the direction of the black stripes on each nail.

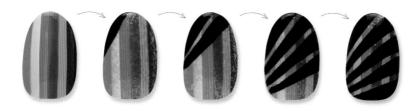

MULTICOLOURED CHEVRONS

Clear crystals add sparkling jewelled detail to these vibrant "V"-shaped tips.

YOU WILL NEED:

nail polish colours in green, orange, pink and bright blue, striping brush, clear crystals and nail glue, plus base coat and top coat.

1   After prepping the nails and applying a base coat, paint all 10 nails with two coats of green polish. Leave to dry.

2   Using a striping brush dipped in orange polish, paint a diagonal line from the right-hand side of each nail at the cuticle to the left-hand side of the tip and fill in with orange.

3   Using a striping brush dipped in pink polish, paint a line from the left-hand side of the cuticle to the centre of the nail to meet the orange, creating a

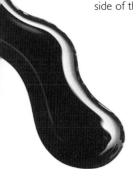

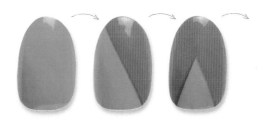

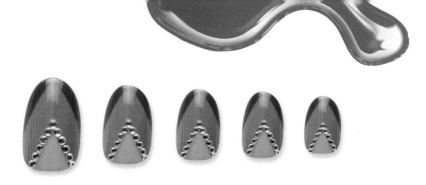

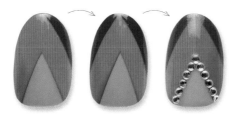

green triangle at the cuticle end of the nail. Then paint a pink line from the tip of the green triangle to the centre of the tip of the nail. Fill in the left-hand side with pink.

4   Using a striping brush dipped in bright blue polish, paint a diagonal tip on the right-hand side of the nail, followed by a matching one on the left-hand side, to create a chevron French tip.

5   When dry, seal with a top coat.

6   Stick crystals along the green chevron "V" formation. Leave to set.

7   Seal with a top coat.

BLUE AZTEC

This summer must-have print can be your firm festival favourite — try different colourways on press-on nails to take with you.

YOU WILL NEED:

nail art pens or polish colours in pastel blue, white and black, striping brush, fine detail brush and dotting tool (if not using pens), plus base coat and top coat.

1 After prepping the nails and applying a base coat, paint two coats of pastel blue on all 10 nails. Leave to dry.

2 Using a striping brush dipped in white polish, paint a band of white across the centre of the nail.

3 Outline the band with two thin black lines using a striping brush dipped in black polish.

4 Paint a thinner black line next to the outer lines.

5 Using a black nail art pen or a fine detail brush dipped in black polish, paint downwards-facing triangles from the thin line to the centre of the white band.

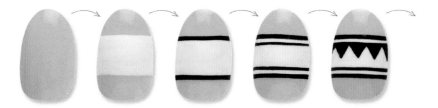

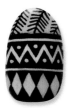

6   Repeat from the other thin line, with the triangles facing upwards, leaving a small white gap between.

7   From the outside line closest to the cuticle, paint more triangles along the line to halfway down the pastel blue.

8   From the cuticle line, paint triangles that meet point-to-point with the other triangles.

9   Paint black "feathers" at the tip: draw a curved line first, then diagonal lines either side all the way along the line. Then add two feathers on either side.

10 Using a white nail art pen or a dotting tool dipped in white polish, add dots to the triangles inside the white band. When dry, apply a top coat.

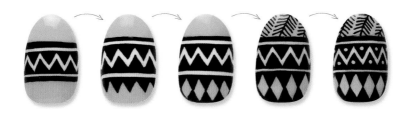

PINK DIAMOND

A simple diamond shape makes a big impact in bright pink, silver and black.

YOU WILL NEED:

nail polish colours in hot pink, silver and black, striping brush, plus base coat and top coat.

1   After prepping the nails and applying a base coat, paint all 10 nails with two coats of hot pink polish. Leave to dry.

2   Using a striping brush dipped in silver polish, draw a silver diagonal line from the left centre of the nail to the centre tip and fill in.

3   Repeat on the other side to create a chevron silver tip.

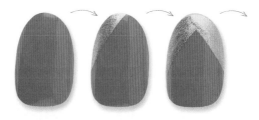

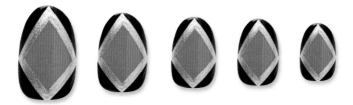

---

4   Repeat at the cuticle end, so that you have another silver chevron at the base and a pink diamond shape in the centre of the nail.

5   Using a striping brush dipped in black polish, paint two more diagonal lines at the cuticle end, on top of the silver, from left to centre and right to centre, leaving a V-shape of silver still visible.

6   Repeat at the tip, so that you now have a chevron black French tip with an outline of silver around the pink diamond.

7   When dry, seal with a top coat.

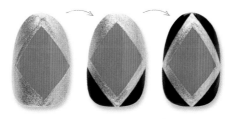

AFRICAN BATIK

Take it slow with this multi-layered effect. You will need patience to work your way through all the layers but the results are incredible.

YOU WILL NEED:

nail art pens or polish colours in lime green, black, pastel pink and hot pink, striping brush and fine detail brush (if not using pens), plus base coat and top coat.

1 After prepping the nails and applying a base coat, paint two coats of lime green polish to all 10 nails. Leave to dry.

2 Using a striping brush dipped in black polish, paint three diagonal lines across the nail, making sure they are spread evenly apart. Start the first line at the centre of the cuticle end of the nail to give you a guide.

3 Paint black diagonal lines going the other way, to create a diamond fishnet effect. You should have a cross going through the centre of the nail.

4 Using a pastel pink nail art pen or fine detail brush dipped in pastel pink polish, paint semicircles in the right-hand corner of each diamond.

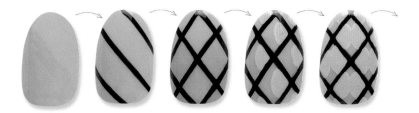

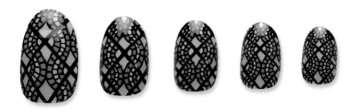

5   Paint pastel pink semicircles in the left-hand corner of each diamond.
    The semicircles should sit back-to-back in the diamond shape.

6   Using a hot pink nail art pen or fine detail brush dipped in hot pink polish,
    draw two lines on top of the pastel pink polish, following the shape of the
    semicircle to create a wavy pattern. Repeat on all the semicircles.

7   Once the pink is dry, use a black nail art pen or fine detail brush dipped
    in black polish to outline the pattern you have made and add lines between
    the pale pink and the hot pink.

8   Add small black lines through each pink stripe to create a mosaic effect.

9   When dry, seal with a top coat.

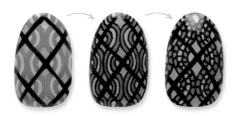

PINK STRIPES

You can't go wrong with classic stripes! Vary the width or change the colours for different effects.

YOU WILL NEED:

nail polish colours in sheer pink, hot pink, red and burgundy, striping brush, plus base coat and top coat.

1 After prepping the nails and applying a base coat, paint all 10 nails with two coats of sheer pink polish. Leave to dry.

2 Using a striping brush dipped in hot pink polish, paint a pink line at the cuticle end of the nail and fill in.

3 Using a striping brush dipped in red polish, paint a line at the tip of the nail and fill in.

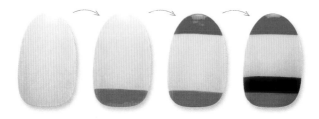

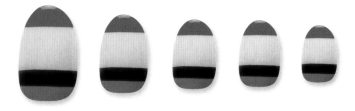

4 Using a striping brush dipped in burgundy polish, paint a thick line above the hot pink.

5 Leave to dry, then seal with a top coat.

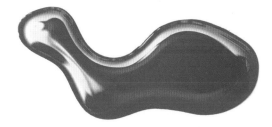

TOP TIP

• *To keep lines looking neat and consistent, thoroughly clean your striping brush with nail polish remover between line placements. A build-up of polish on the brush can lead to thicker, wobbly-looking lines.*

SURFBOARD

Get into the California beach vibe with this boogie board design.

YOU WILL NEED:

nail polish colours in bright/neon orange, light blue, dark blue, black and neon pink, striping brush, white nail art pen, plus base coat and top coat.

1   After prepping the nails and applying a base coat, paint all 10 nails with two coats of bright/neon orange polish. Leave to dry.

2   Using a striping brush dipped in light blue polish, paint two thick vertical lines, so the nail is divided into three equal orange strips with blue lines between the orange.

3   Using a striping brush dipped in dark blue polish, paint lines on the outer edge of the light blue lines. Make sure you leave the orange strip in the centre of the nail.

4   With a striping brush dipped in black polish, paint black lines on the outer edge of the dark blue lines.

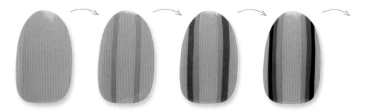

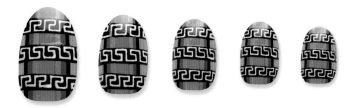

5   Cover the strips of orange on the outer edges of the nail using a striping brush dipped in neon pink polish.

6   Use a striping brush dipped in black polish to paint a thick band of black horizontally across the centre of the nail.

7   Paint two more black bands of the same thickness above and below the first band.

8   When dry, use a white nail art pen to draw the pattern on the top and bottom black bands. Start by drawing upside-down "L" shapes along the black line, then join them up so that the pattern looks like a Greek key design.

9   Draw the Greek key design on the middle black band, but this time have the pattern face the opposite way.

10 Leave to dry, then seal with a top coat.

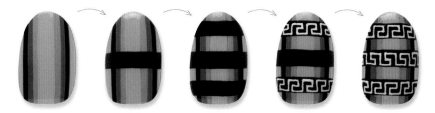

ART DECO

This sun-ray Deco design in pink glitter creates the perfect 1920s flapper look.

YOU WILL NEED:

nail polish colours in pink glitter and black, striping brush, plus base coat and top coat.

1   After prepping the nails and applying a base coat, paint all 10 nails with two coats of pink glitter polish. Leave to dry.

2   Using a striping brush dipped in black polish, paint an elongated triangle section from the tip of the nail over to the left, extending to just above the cuticle line.

3   Paint another black triangle section to the right of the first, making sure to leave a thin gap of pink glitter in between.

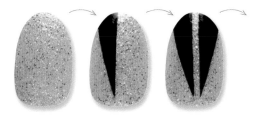

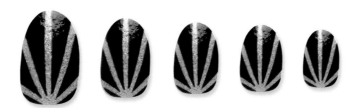

4 Paint a slightly wider triangle shape next to this, leaving the same-sized gap of pink in between.

5 Paint another black triangle section on the left-hand side, with the same-sized gap of pink in between. The design should start looking like a "sun-ray" design.

6 Where there is pink space at the cuticle, fill in with black stripes on both sides.

7 When dry, seal with a top coat.

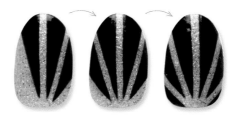

RETRO GRAPHIC

A Mondrian-inspired pattern is worked in hot vibrant colours but you could opt for primary colours of blue, red and yellow.

YOU WILL NEED:

nail polish colours in lime green, orange, hot pink and black, striping brush, plus base coat and top coat.

1   After prepping the nails and applying a base coat, paint all 10 nails with two coats of lime green polish. Leave to dry.

2   Using a striping brush dipped in orange polish, paint a vertical line on the left-hand side of each nail, about one-quarter of the way across the nail, and fill in.

3   Using a striping brush dipped in hot pink polish, split the green in half by painting a square of pink at the base of the nail.

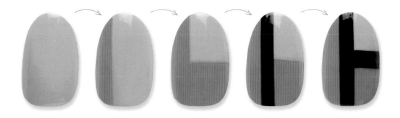

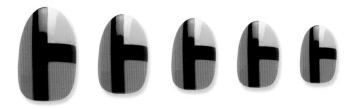

4   Outline the orange strip with a thick line of black using a striping brush dipped in black polish.

5   Outline where the green and pink meet with a thick line of black.

6   When dry, apply a top coat.

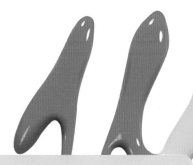

TOP TIP

• You don't need to be too perfect when painting the colour sections as the black will cover the lines that meet anyway!

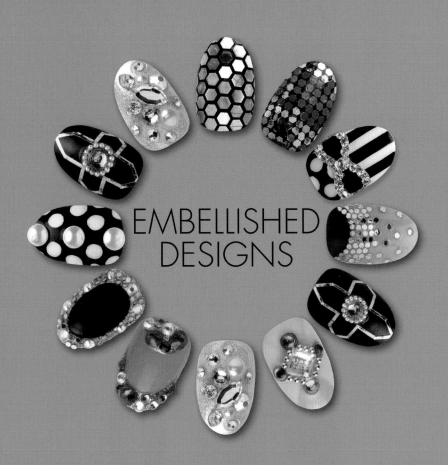

EMBELLISHED
DESIGNS

DISCO BALL

Holographic hexagonal discs are used to create a mirrored mosaic design.

YOU WILL NEED:

nail polish in black, small stick-on hexagonal foil discs, cocktail stick (toothpick) or dotting tool, stork (embroidery) scissors, plus base coat and top coat.

1   Prep and apply a base coat. Paint two coats of black polish to all 10 nails. Do not allow to dry.

2   Pour the hexagonal discs onto a piece of card or sheet of paper. Using a cocktail stick (toothpick) or dotting tool, pick up and place a vertical row of discs down the centre of the nail, from the tip to the cuticle. Make sure to leave a small gap of black between each disc.

3   Add another vertical row of discs next to the one you have just made – the hexagons should fit in the gaps like a honeycomb. Remember to leave a small gap of black between each disc.

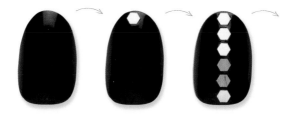

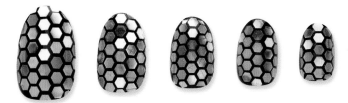

4   Continue making vertical rows of hexagonal discs in the honeycomb formation over the nail until it is covered. If the black polish has dried and the discs won't stick, use a top coat to wet the nail as you go.

5   If there are small gaps at the side or the tip of the nail where a whole hexagon won't fit, cut a disc in half and place it on the nail to fill the gaps. This will ensure that every part of the nail is covered.

6   When dry, seal with a top coat.

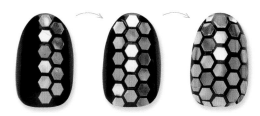

SATURDAY NIGHT FEVER

This variation on the disco ball uses foil glitter pieces to provide a dazzling effect.

YOU WILL NEED:

nail polish in black, foil glitter discs in rainbow colours, cocktail stick (toothpick), plus base coat and top coat.

1   Prep and apply a base coat. Paint two coats of black nail polish on all 10 nails. Do not allow to dry.

2   Pour some of the glitter discs onto a piece of card or sheet of paper.

3   Using a cocktail stick (toothpick), pick out pieces of gold glitter. Place a row of gold on the tip end of the nail; depending on the size of the nail, make one or two neat horizontal rows – the pieces should sit neatly next to each other with a small gap in between, so that the black is visible.

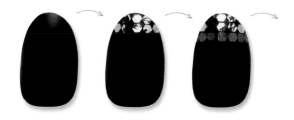

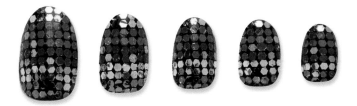

4   Pick out pieces of red glitter and place them in a row below the gold.

5   Next add a row a of pink glitter.

6   Add two rows of mixed light and dark blue glitter pieces below the pink row.

7   Place two rows of silver glitter pieces below the blue rows.

8   Finally, add a green glitter row below the silver.

9   Seal with a top coat.

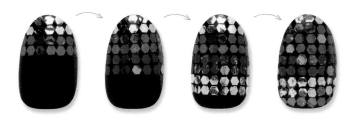

MONOCHROME BOWS

Add sparkling detail with diamond bows on top of black-and-white spots and stripes.

YOU WILL NEED:

nail polish colours in white and black, striping brush, fine detail brush, large dotting tool, nail glue, diamond-encrusted nail art bows, 3D flat-backed pearls (optional), plus base and top coat.

1   After prepping the nails and applying a base coat, paint all 10 nails with two coats of white polish. Leave to dry.

2   Paint a large half moon at the cuticle end with a striping brush or fine detail brush dipped in black polish.

3   Using a striping brush and black polish, paint a thick vertical stripe from the centre top of the half moon to the centre tip of the nail. Then paint the rest of the vertical black stripes.

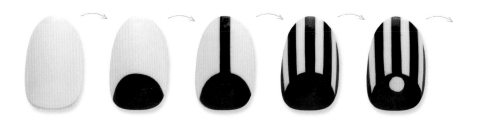

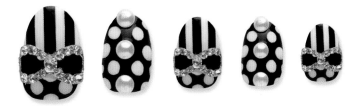

4 Using a large dotting tool dipped in white polish, paint a white spot inside the top of the black half moon.

5 Add more white spots to the half moon, one below the first spot and two in the spaces either side.

6 When the spots are dry, apply a top coat to all the nails.

7 When the top coat is dry, place a little spot of nail glue at the top of the half moon and place a diamond-encrusted bow on top. Press down until the bow is stuck firmly to the nail.

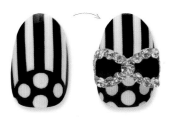

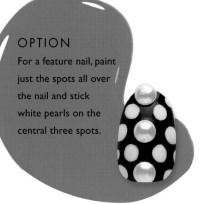

OPTION

For a feature nail, paint just the spots all over the nail and stick white pearls on the central three spots.

MOSAIC MOONS

Sequins are used to stunning effect in a design that has a hint of Art Deco about it.

YOU WILL NEED:

nail polish colours in nude and dark blue, fine detail brush, gold flatstone nail art sequins, cocktail stick (toothpick), plus base coat and top coat.

1   After prepping the nails and applying a base coat, paint all 10 nails with two coats of nude polish. Leave to dry.

2   At each cuticle end, paint a half moon using a fine detail brush dipped in dark blue polish.

3   When the dark blue is dry, paint on a top coat – it's best to do this one nail at a time, so that the top coat is still wet enough to apply the flatstones in the next step.

4   While the top coat is still wet, apply a line of gold flatstone sequins around the half moon using a cocktail stick (toothpick).

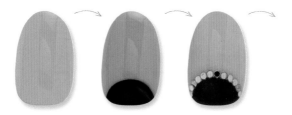

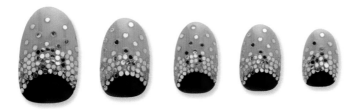

5 Add another line of gold flatstones directly above the first.

6 Apply two more lines of flatstones until you have four in total. If the top coat dries while you are applying the flatstones, apply a little more top coat where needed in order for the flatstones to stick.

7 Above the last line of flatstones apply more flatstones, but leave some nude spaces between them.

8 In the remaining nude section, scatter gold flatstones in a gradient effect towards the tip.

9 Add a final top coat to seal everything in.

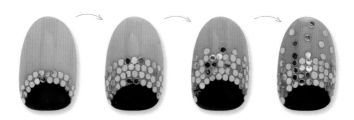

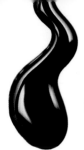

GOTHIC CROSSES

This jewelled design will give an edgy embellishment to your look.

YOU WILL NEED:

nail polish in black, nail glue, tweezers, coloured nail art crystals, cocktail stick (toothpick), tiny silver bullion beads, stork (embroidery) scissors, gold nail art striping tape, plus base coat and top coat.

1   After prepping and applying a base coat, paint all 10 nails with two thin coats of black nail polish.

2   In the centre of the nail, add a drop of nail glue and then, using tweezers, apply a coloured crystal. Lightly push it down into the glue so that it sticks.

3   Add a little more nail glue around the crystal. Using a cocktail stick (toothpick), push tiny silver bullion beads into the glue around the crystal.

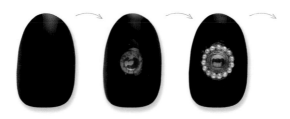

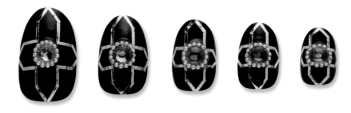

4   Cut two small pieces of gold striping tape and place them vertically above the crystal.

5   Repeat step 4 vertically and horizontally around the crystal to create a criss-cross pattern. There should be eight pieces of gold tape in total.

6   Cut two more pieces of gold tape and place on the top of the two vertical strips towards the nail tip, creating an upside-down "V".

7   Add "V" shapes to the three other branches of the cross. Make sure the gold tape is stuck securely by pressing lightly with a cocktail stick.

8   Finish with a top coat to seal.

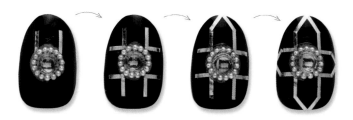

PASTEL HARLEQUIN

The brightly coloured crystals really bring this pastel pattern to life. Try customizing each nail differently for a fun eye-catching effect.

YOU WILL NEED:

nail polish colours in pastel pink, pastel purple, pastel blue and pastel yellow, striping brush, nail glue, diamond-shaped clear crystals, cuticle stick, coloured crystals, gold bullion beads, plus base coat and top coat.

1 After prepping the nails and applying a base coat, apply two coats of pastel pink polish to each nail.

2 Using a striping brush dipped in pastel purple polish, divide the nail into two diagonally, from tip to cuticle, and fill in the top half with the purple.

3 Using a striping brush dipped in pastel blue polish, divide the nail in half again from the other side of the nail, left cuticle to right tip. The nail should now be split into three coloured sections.

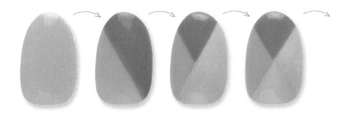

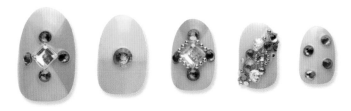

4 Using a striping brush dipped in pastel yellow polish, divide the nail into four sections by splitting the blue section in half diagonally. Fill it in. You should now have four triangular sections. When dry, seal with a top coat.

5 Add a small dot of nail glue to the centre of the nail and add a diamond-shaped crystal using a cuticle stick. Press down slightly until firmly in place.

6 Above the top point of the diamond, add another small drop of nail glue and place a coloured crystal in the glue. At each point of the diamond, apply glue and a different-coloured crystal.

7 Add a little more glue around the main crystal and apply gold bullion beads in a line all the way around the diamond.

8 When dry, apply another top coat to seal the crystals.

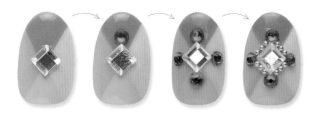

TIARA TIPS

This beautiful embellishment is perfect for a fairytale bride.

YOU WILL NEED:

nail polish in metallic/glittery white, nail glue, marquee-shaped crystals, tweezers, cuticle stick, rose-coloured crystals, aurora borealis crystals, 3D pear-shaped crystals in clear and rose, smaller nail art crystals and pearls, plus base coat and top coat.

1   After prepping the nails and applying a base coat, paint all 10 nails with two coats of metallic/glittery white nail polish.

2   Place a dot of nail glue or top coat (nail glue will hold the bigger stones better) in the centre of the nail and apply a marquee-shaped crystal to the glue. Press down firmly with a cuticle stick.

3   On either side of the marquee crystal, apply two more dots of nail glue and place a rose-coloured crystal on one side and an aurora borealis-coloured crystal on the other.

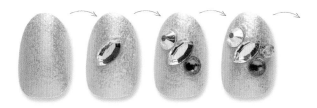

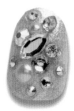

4 Place another dot of glue above the rose stone and apply a 3D pear-shaped crystal, holding it in place with a cuticle stick until firmly stuck down.

5 Add more dots of glue and sit two pearls into it, above and below the marquee crystal.

6 Add more glue above the 3D pear and apply a 3D rose-coloured pear crystal, holding it in place with a cuticle stick until firmly stuck down.

7 In the space to the left of the cluster of crystals you have created, add dots of glue in a gradient effect. Place smaller crystals and pearls on the glue dots, so that you have a burst of crystals radiating out from the main cluster of diamonds towards the sides of the nail, tip and cuticle.

8 Finish with a top coat, but make sure to get into and around the stones with the brush!

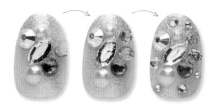

SAPPHIRE MOONS

*Blue stones add glamour and sparkle
to an elegant nude base.*

YOU WILL NEED:

nail polish colours in nude and gold glitter, striping brush, nail glue, crystals in diamond, light blue and dark blue in different sizes, plus base coat and top coat.

1   After prepping the nails and applying a base coat, paint all 10 nails with two coats of nude polish.

2   Using a striping brush dipped in gold glitter polish, paint a curved French tip.

3   Paint the outline of a half moon in a thick band of gold glitter.

4   Add a mix of diamond, light blue and dark blue crystals to the nails at the half moon using a little nail glue or top coat.

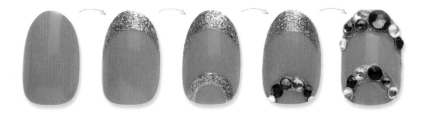

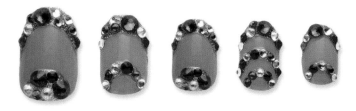

5 Apply a little nail glue to the tip of the nail and then place different sizes and shades of blue and diamond crystals in a cluster at the tip.

6 Paint a top coat over all the nails, making sure to get right into the sides of the stones.

For the Full Set: On some nails, paint a third gold curve line in the middle of the nail and stick on clusters of blue and diamond crystals in different sizes using nail glue or top coat. Alternatively, paint some solid gold glitter half moons and stick on clusters of blue and diamond crystals in the same way.

TOP TIPS

• *Use a nail adhesive that states it dries clear. Some adhesives can leave a frosty white residue when dry, which can ruin the look of the design.*

• *If you get any glue or polish on the embellishments, remove it with a brush dipped in a little nail polish remover before you apply the top coat.*

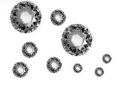

BLACK ORLOV

The Black Orlov is a beautiful black diamond. Recreate your own precious stones and flaunt them on your fingertips.

YOU WILL NEED:

nail polish colours in black and gold, striping brush, small diamond crystals, gold flatstone sequins, nail glue, plus base coat and top coat.

1   After prepping the nails and applying a base coat, paint all 10 nails with two coats of black polish.

2   Using a striping brush dipped in gold polish, paint a thick outline all around the edge of the nails.

3   Fix four diamond crystals using a dot of nail glue or top coat on the gold outline, one at the tip, one at the cuticle end and one on either side of the nail.

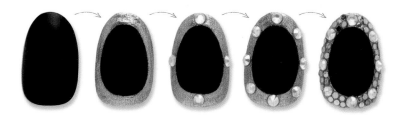

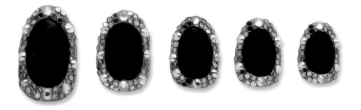

4 Add four more crystals, one between each of the crystals you have just applied, so that you have eight crystals evenly placed inside the outline around the nail.

5 In the spaces between the crystals, apply a little top coat and place small gold flatstone sequins to cover the rest of the gold outline.

6 Apply a top coat over all the nails to seal.

TOP TIPS

• Use a damp wooden manicure stick to pick up and place crystals easily – or use tweezers, a dotting tool or even the tip of a pencil.

• Apply the nail adhesive in stages, one nail at a time, as it can dry very quickly.

• Don't apply too much glue or your finished design may show unwelcome blobs and bumps.

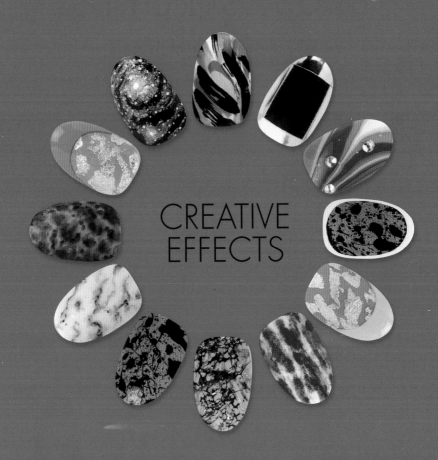

CREATIVE
EFFECTS

BRUSHSTROKES

*Modern Art was the inspiration
for this abstract, painterly effect.*

YOU WILL NEED:

*nail polish colours in white, yellow, blue, red and black, fine detail brush, plus base coat
and top coat.*

1   After prepping and applying a base coat, apply two coats of white paint to all
    10 nails. Leave to dry.

2   Dip the brush into the yellow polish and wipe off the excess on the side of
    the bottle. Wipe off more polish with a piece of tissue. The brush needs to be
    quite dry to create the brushstroke effect. Paint random brushstrokes across
    the surface of the nail, adding more or less polish to the brush as necessary.

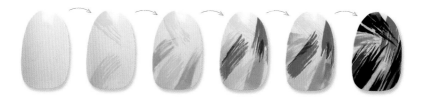

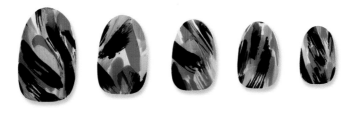

3. Repeat with the green polish, making randomly placed brushstrokes. Overlap the colours, too.

4. Repeat with the red, then the blue and finally the black polish. You want to be able to see some of the white base peeking through.

5. When dry, seal with a top coat and enjoy your work of art!

TOP TIP

• The brushstroke effect works best with minimal colour on the brush, so make sure you wipe off any excess on a tissue or piece of paper before applying. If your brushstrokes haven't turned out as well as you'd hoped, you can paint into them with a fine detail brush to enhance the brush effect.

TURQUOISE STONE

*Try out this simple marbling technique to create
a beautiful precious-stone design.*

YOU WILL NEED:

*nail polish colours in turquoise and black, small bowl filled with water, hairspray,
wooden cocktail sticks, cotton buds (Q-tips), nail polish remover, nail polish in gold
(or gold nail art foil and adhesive), plus base coat and top coat.*

1 After prepping the nails and applying a base coat, apply two coats of
turquoise polish to all 10 nails. Leave to dry.

2 Take a small bowl filled with water and place a drop of black polish into the
water using the brush in the polish bottle. One drop of black is enough, but if
you want the design to be darker you can add another drop of black.

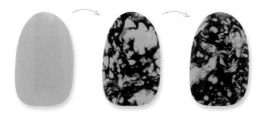

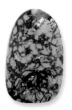

3 As the polish spreads out into the water, spray the surface of the water with hairspray. You will see the polish disperse and create a veiny pattern on the water.

4 Choose the area of the pattern in the water that you want your design to be and position your nail over it. Dip your nail into the water and use a cocktail stick (toothpick) or cotton bud (Q-tip) to pick up the leftover polish on the surface of the water around your finger before you remove your nail from the water.

5 Clean off the polish on your finger and cuticle with a cotton bud or tidy-up brush dipped in nail polish remover. Complete all 10 nails.

6 Once the nails are dry, use a brush dipped in gold nail polish (or use gold nail art foil and adhesive) to add gold fleck detailing on the "stone" pattern. If using the gold foil, paint the glue where you want the gold to go, leave the glue to dry and then rub the gold foil on top.

7 Finish with a top coat to seal.

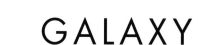

GALAXY

Clouds and comet swirls create a little universe on each nail!

YOU WILL NEED:

nail polish colours in black, silver/pearly white, blue glitter, metallic purple, gold and white, fine detail brush, plus base coat and top coat.

1 After prepping the nails and applying a base coat, paint all 10 nails with two coats of black polish. Leave to dry.

2 Using a small detail brush dipped in a silver/pearly white polish, paint a dot in the centre of the nail about one-quarter of the way from the tip. Pat the polish with your finger to blend it a little so it looks "cloud-like" and not so solid. Then add another smaller dot on top.

3 Using the same colour, draw a curved line around this central spot. Pat down with your finger to blend out a little. Paint swirls above and around the central "cloud", patting to blend.

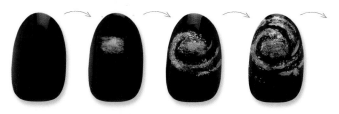

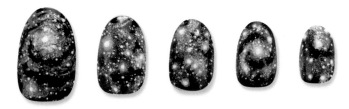

4   Continue painting more swirls below the cloud, this time adding some smaller dot/cloud shapes underneath. Pat down to make the colour more translucent.

5   Using blue glitter polish and a small detail brush, add dashes of blue to the swirls and around the central cloud. Don't overdo it – just add little glimpses of colour and blend with the brush or your fingertip to make the colour soft.

6   Using metallic purple and gold polishes, add swirls or dots around the central cloud and to the smaller clouds. Build up the colour in stages, blending all the time. Avoid completely covering the first pearl-coloured clouds and swirls.

7   Add a white dot in the centre of each cloud and tiny little dots inside the swirls. Scatter a few into the black to give that galaxy starburst effect. Do not paint your dots too big – the bigger the dot, the clunkier the design looks! Be light and paint delicate dots for the true galaxy effect!

8   When dry, seal with a top coat.

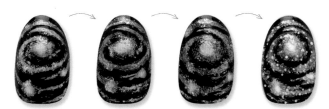

GOLD FRAME

Make a statement with this chic metallic border design, originally created for a fashion shoot with an Egyptian theme!

YOU WILL NEED:

nail polish in dark inky blue, sticky-back gold nail art foil, plus base coat and top coat.

1   After prepping and applying a base coat, paint all 10 nails with two coats of dark inky blue polish. Leave to dry.

2   Cut out two strips of gold nail art foil, both the same width, to fit down the sidewalls of your nail. Place it over the nail to check that you have cut the correct size before applying.

3   Then fit one of the gold strips in place on the left-hand edge of the nail and press down. The gold foil has a sticky back so it should stick without using any top coat or glue. If there is overhang at the tip, file it off by filing in a downward motion.

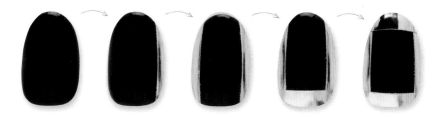

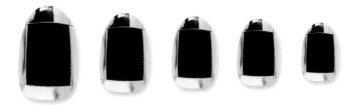

4 Fit the other gold strip to the right-hand edge of the nail and file off any overhang at the tip.

5 Now cut a piece of gold foil to fit at the cuticle end. Cut a strip the same width as the others but cut it into a curve to fit smoothly into the base at the cuticle. Check the fit before pressing it down to stick.

6 Cut another gold strip for the nail tip to the same width as the others. You don't have to be as precise with this one, as once you have stuck it on, you can file off any overhang.

7 Apply a top coat to seal in the gold foil.

TOP TIP

• *Before you start painting, place the gold foil over each nail to judge the size and curve of each cuticle and side wall. Cut to shape and set aside in nail order on your work station while you paint the inky blue base. Sizing the gold foil before you paint means you won't be tempted to do it while the base is still wet and smudge the colour.*

CARRARA MARBLE

Inspired by Italian carrara marble, this design gives a sculptural feel to the fingertips.

YOU WILL NEED:

nail polish colours in white, light grey, dark grey and black, aluminium foil, nail polish remover, fine detail brush, plus base coat and top coat.

1 After prepping and applying a base coat, paint all 10 nails with two coats of white polish. Leave to dry.

2 Pour a little light grey polish onto a piece of aluminium foil and mix with a little polish remover. Paint this mixture in "vein–like" marble markings across the nails using a small detail brush.

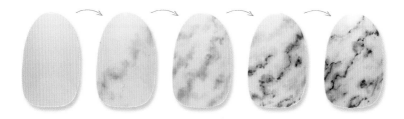

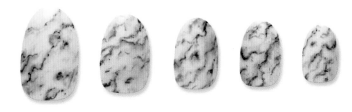

3   Add more grey polish/polish remover mixture to the veins to build up the colour, bit by bit. Add more grey to your mix to make some parts of the marble "veins" darker.

4   Add darker grey detailing to some areas of the "veins" using a small detail brush dipped in dark grey polish, building up the effect as you work.

5   Using a small detail brush and black polish, add fine lines inside the grey "veins".

6   When dry, apply a top coat to seal.

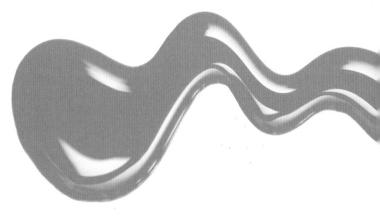

ACID WASH

Wear a stripped-back acid-wash effect on your nails as well as your jeans!

YOU WILL NEED:

nail polish colours in dark blue and white, cotton buds (Q-tips), nail polish remover, plus base coat and top coat.

1   After prepping and applying a base coat, apply two coats of dark blue polish to all 10 nails.

2   Once the blue is dry, paint a thin coat of white polish over the top.

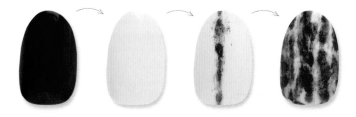

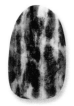

3 When the white is dry, dip a cotton bud in nail polish remover and dab the excess off on a tissue. Roll the cotton bud in a vertical direction back and forth on the nail to remove some of the white and reveal the blue underneath.

4 Continue rolling in lines and dashes with the cotton bud, adding more nail polish remover if necessary. The blue should be revealed and the nail polish remover should blend the blue into the white a little, creating that acid-wash denim effect.

5 Finish with a top coat to seal.

TOP TIP

• *Be very gentle when rolling the cotton bud over the polish as you don't want to take too much away and reveal a bare nail underneath!*

PSYCHEDELIC NAILS

Go "hippy chic" with this hypnotic multicoloured effect, perfect for hazy, summer days.

YOU WILL NEED:

nail polish colours in white, red, orange, yellow, pink, light blue and dark blue (as many as you like!), small bowl filled with water, wooden cocktail sticks, nail polish remover, cotton buds (Q-tips) or a tidy-up brush, small clear crystals, nail glue, plus base coat and top coat.

I   After prepping and applying a base coat, paint all 10 nails with two coats of white polish and leave to dry. The white is a great base colour as it really brings out the colours of the water marbling.

TOP TIP

• *Before you begin, cover the fingers with masking tape, leaving only the nail visible. This ensures that only the nail will pick up colour and you won't have to clean up the surrounding skin afterwards. My preferred method, however, is to cover the surrounding skin with a coat of peel-off base coat, which you can simply peel and discard at the end.. Easy peasy!*

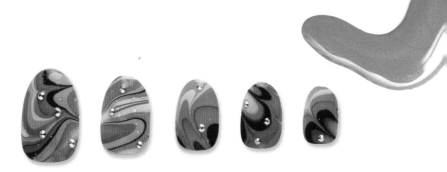

2 Take a small bowl filled with water and add a drop of red polish. Then add a drop of orange, then yellow, pink, light blue and dark blue all on top of one another to create colour rings. You can add as many colours as you like.

3 Swirl the colours by running a cocktail stick through them. Start from the middle of the colour drop and drag outwards – starting from the outer edge tends to mess up the design. Wipe off the polish from the cocktail stick each time you place it in the water to make a swirl, to avoid transferring colour where you don't want it.

4 Choose the area of the pattern in the water that you want for your design and position your nail over it. Dip your nail into the water and use a cocktail stick or cotton bud to pick up the leftover polish on the surface of the water around your finger before you remove your nail from the water.

5 Clean off the polish on your finger and cuticle with a cotton bud or tidy-up brush dipped in remover. Repeat the process until all 10 nails are complete and leave to dry.

6 Using a little nail glue or top coat, stick on a few crystals, scattered over the design.

7 Apply a top coat to seal.

SPLATTER PAINT

A super-easy nail design that makes a big impact. Make sure you cover your work surfaces as it can get a little messy!

YOU WILL NEED:

nail polish colours in hot pink, black and white, aluminum foil, drinking straw, cotton buds (Q-tips) or a fine detail brush, nail polish remover, striping brush, plus base coat and top coat.

1   After prepping and applying a base coat, paint all 10 nails with two coats of hot pink. Leave to dry.

2   Dab a blob of black polish on to a piece of aluminium foil. Take a straw and dip the end into the polish. When you dip the straw into the black polish make sure you pick up enough polish to completely cover the straw hole - you'll find it will splatter better.

3   Positioning the straw over one nail, blow into the other end of the straw with a short sharp burst of breath, so that the polish splatters across the nails. Pick up more polish and repeat until you have splatters on each nail.

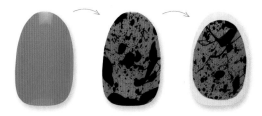

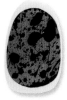

4 You're going to have some black polish on the surrounding skin and cuticle, no matter how careful you were. Clean the bulk of this off using a cotton bud dipped in nail polish remover. Then, using a fine detail brush dipped in nail polish remover, remove any stray polish closer to the cuticle or nail (see also Top Tips below). You can also use protect the skin from colour with masking tape or use peel-off base coat (see Glitter, page 22).

5 When the black splatter is dry, outline the nails with a white border using a striping brush dipped in white polish.

6 When dry, finish with a top coat to seal.

TOP TIPS

• *Practise your splattering on a piece of paper first to find the method that works best for you.*

• *To avoid as much polish going onto the skin as possible try blowing away from the finger towards the tip and always make sure your work surfaces are covered with newspaper.*

TORTOISESHELL

The beautiful mottled appearance of tortoiseshell is here replicated by blending cloud-like shapes together across the surface of the nail.

YOU WILL NEED:

nail polish colours in mustard yellow, orange, reddish brown, brown and dark brown, aluminium foil, nail polish remover, fine detail brush, plus base coat and top coat.

1   After prepping the nails and applying a base coat, paint two coats of mustard yellow polish on all 10 nails. Leave to dry.

2   Add a few drops of orange polish to a sheet of aluminium foil and mix with a little nail polish remover. Paint the orange/remover mix in irregular "cloud-like" shapes across the nail using a small detail brush.

3   Mix some more orange polish with remover, but this time add more orange to make a slightly stronger pigment. Apply to the inside of the irregular "cloud" shapes to build up the colour.

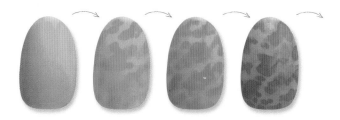

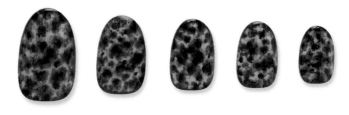

4   Mix a few drops of reddish brown polish with some nail polish remover on aluminium foil and add this on top of the orange shapes. Do not completely cover the orange but leave the orange peeking through in places.

5   Mix more reddish brown polish with remover to make a darker brown mix and add to the middle of the brown shapes you've just created. Then repeat with an even darker brown colour, leaving the lighter shades visible around it.

6   Build up the brown with darker brown polish mixed with nail polish remover. Use to add some irregular dashes and spots to the design.

7   Add a very dark brown polish (not mixed with any remover) to the centre of the irregular shapes, dashes and dots and outline the whole nail to create a dark brown border. When dry, apply a top coat to seal.

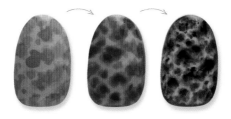

FLECKED GOLD LEAF

The mix of bold bright colours combined with the ornate gold leaf really makes this nail design pop.

YOU WILL NEED:

nail polish colours in bright purple and hot pink, gold leaf foil, wooden cuticle stick, cotton bud (Q-tip) or fine detail brush, striping brush, plus base coat and top coat.

1 After prepping and applying a base coat, paint all 10 nails with purple polish.

2 When the polish has dried a little but is still tacky, take a small piece of gold leaf foil and place onto the nail with a cuticle stick and smooth it down lightly into the polish with a cotton bud or brush. If the polish is too wet, the gold leaf can become crumpled and look untidy.

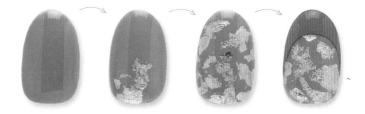

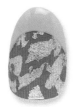

3 Apply gold leaf randomly all over the nail in the same way, making sure the purple is still visible between.

4 Using a striping brush, paint a hot pink French tip.

5 When dry, apply a top coat to seal.

For the Full Set: Alternate the nails and tips with different colours!

TOP TIPS

• If you haven't pressed the gold leaf down properly, it might be tricky for you to paint a clean, neat French tip. You can rectify this by applying a top coat over the gold leaf nail first and then, when dry, you'll have a smoother base to paint a French tip on top.

• You can paint your French tip first before applying the gold leaf if you prefer, but this will risk getting the gold leaf on the tip.

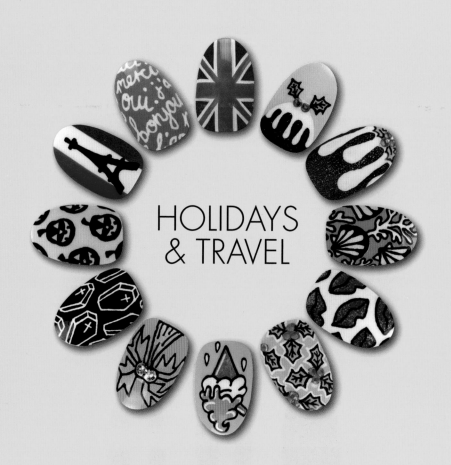

HOLIDAYS
& TRAVEL

UNION JACK

*Rule Britannia with this patriotic flag design —
ideal for a tourist's trip to London !*

YOU WILL NEED:

nail polish colours in blue glitter, red and white, striping brush, plus base coat and top coat.

1 Prep and apply a base coat. Apply two coats of blue glitter polish on all 10 nails. Leave to dry.

2 Using a striping brush dipped in white polish, paint a white strip vertically down the middle of the nail.

3 Paint a white strip of the same width horizontally across the middle of the nail to create a white cross.

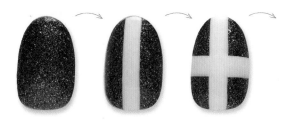

4 Again, with the striping brush dipped in white polish, paint a slightly narrower white strip diagonally across the nail from the top left to the bottom right.

5 Repeat step 4 but paint the strip from the left bottom to the top right. You will now have the basis for a Union Jack flag.

6 Using red glitter polish, paint a cross within the first main white cross, leaving equal strips of white at the edges.

7 Do the same within the diagonal lines, leaving the same amount of white at the edges.

8 When dry, seal with a top coat.

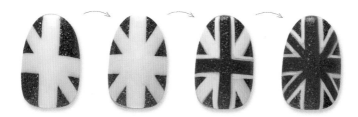

STARS & STRIPES

Rock the stars and stripes this Fourth of July with red, white and blue at your fingertips!

YOU WILL NEED:

nail art pens or polish colours in white, red and blue, striping brush and fine detail brush (if not using pens), plus base coat and top coat.

1 After prepping and applying a base coat, paint all 10 nails with two coats of white polish. Leave to dry.

2 Using a striping brush dipped in red polish, paint a thick vertical line down the middle of the nail.

3 Paint two more stripes the same size on either side of the middle stripe, leaving an equally spaced white gap between. Paint more red stripes until the nail is completely striped.

4 Using a striping or detail brush dipped in blue polish, paint a large half moon at the cuticle end of the nail. Leave to dry.

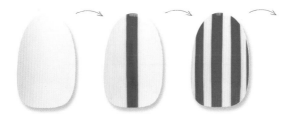

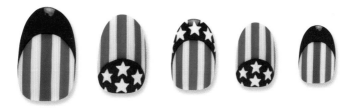

5 Using a white nail art pen or a detail brush and white polish, paint a small star inside the blue half moon at the very top and another directly beneath it.

6 Paint more equally spaced small white stars. To make it look like a continuous overall print, add two little star points at the base of the cuticle.

7 When dry and the set is complete, finish with a top coat!

For the Full Set: Mix up the design with French-tipped stars. Follow steps 1 to 3 but instead of painting a half moon, paint a curved French tip. Leave to dry and paint small white stars. Alternatively, wear full stars-and-stripes designs, or alternate with nails painted with vertical red stripes.

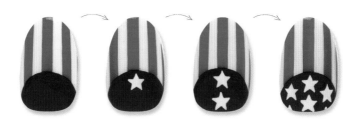

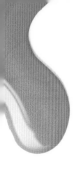

FIGGY PUDDING

The half moon of the nail is the perfect setting for this Christmas pudding on a eye-popping pink background.

YOU WILL NEED:

nail art pens or polish colours in pink, metallic brown, white, light green and dark green, striping brush and fine detail brush (if not using pens), 20 tiny red crystals, wooden cocktail stick (toothpicks) or tweezers, plus base coat and top coat.

1 Prep and apply a base coat. Apply two coats of pink polish on all 10 nails. Leave to dry.

2 Using a striping brush dipped in the metallic brown polish, paint a large half moon in the shape of a Christmas pudding at the cuticle end of the nail.

3 Using a white nail art pen or detail brush dipped in white polish, draw a drippy icing detail to the top of the pudding.

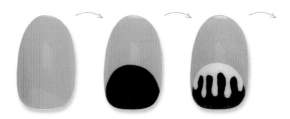

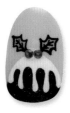

4 Using a light green nail art pen or detail brush dipped in light green polish, draw and fill in two green holly leaf shapes on top of the pudding. Be sure to leave enough space between the leaves for the red crystal holly berries.

5 Using a dark green nail art pen or a detail brush dipped in dark green polish, draw an outline around the holly leaves. Add detail to the leaves by drawing a vertical line down the centre with short dashes adjoining them.

6 Using a cocktail stick or tweezers, dab a little glue or top coat on the nail, between the holly leaves, and stick on two red crystals.

7 When dry, seal with a top coat.

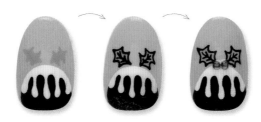

FIGGY PUDDING FRENCH TIPS

A variation on the Figgy Pudding design on the previous pages, this one is the icing on the cake!

YOU WILL NEED:

nail art pens or polish colours in metallic brown and white, light green and dark green, striping brush and fine detail brush (if not using pens), nail glue, 30 tiny red crystals, plus base coat and top coat.

1   After prepping and applying a base coat, apply two coats of metallic brown nail polish to all 10 nails. Leave to dry.

2   Using a striping brush dipped in white nail polish, paint a thin French tip.

3   Using a white nail art pen or detail brush dipped in white polish, paint an "icing" drip shape from the French tip to about halfway down the nail.

4   Add a slightly longer drip to the right of the first drip.

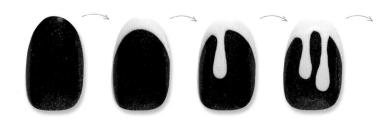

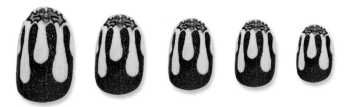

5 Add another long drip to the left of the first drip.

6 Add two smaller drips to the right-hand side. Once the white is dry, take a light green nail art pen or fine detail brush dipped in light green polish and paint two holly leaf shapes at the tip of the nail, making sure to leave space for the red crystal holly berries between them.

7 Outline the leaves with a dark green nail art pen or fine detail brush dipped in dark green polish and add a line through the middle of each leaf.

8 Place a little nail glue or top coat between the leaves and stick on three little red crystals for the berries. Apply a top coat to finish.

For the Full Set: Alternate fingers of Figgy Pudding French Tips with the Figgy Pudding design on pages 164–5.

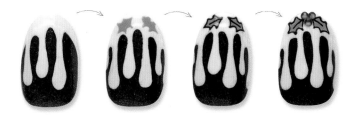

HOLLY PRINT

This holiday holly wrapping-paper-inspired print is perfect for the festive season!

YOU WILL NEED:

nail art pens or polish colours in pastel blue, red, light green and dark green, dotting tool (if not using pens), 90 tiny red crystals, plus base coat and top coat.

1   After preparing your nails and applying a base coat, paint all 10 nails with two coats of pastel blue polish. Leave to dry.

2   Using a red nail art pen or dotting tool dipped in red polish, place two red dots close together randomly on each blue nail. Add another red dot directly above or below in the middle of the first two red dots. These are your three holly berries.

3   Using a light green nail art pen or brush dipped in light green polish, draw a five-pointed holly leaf between the first and the third red dot.

4   Draw on another holly leaf between the second and the third red dot.

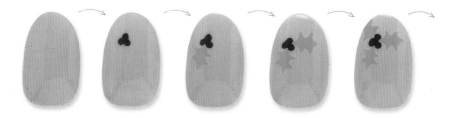

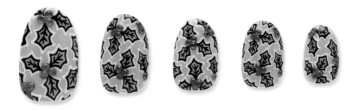

5 And then draw on the third leaf between the first and second red dot.

6 Cover the whole nail in holly berries and leaves, making sure you leave enough of a gap between to outline them.

7 Outline the green leaves with a darker green polish. Add detail to the leaves by drawing a line down the centre of each with two dashes on either side of the line (four dashes in total).

8 Outline the holly leaves with a white nail art pen or detail brush dipped in white polish. The white really makes the design pop!

9 Add a little top coat to the three berries and place three small red crystals on top of the berries. This creates a 3D effect. Finish with a top coat.

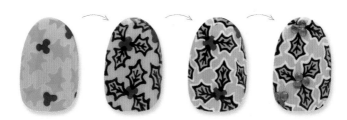

PALM TREES

A hint of gold glitter makes these tropical palms glimmer in the sunshine.

YOU WILL NEED:

nail art pens or polish colours in neon pink, pale gold, gold glitter, light metallic orange, lime green and black, dotting tool and fine detail brush (if not using pens), plus base coat and top coat.

1 After prepping the nails and applying a base coat, apply two coats of neon pink nail polish to all 10 nails. Leave to dry.

2 Using a dotting tool dipped in a light gold polish, apply two dots sitting together just above the middle of the nail.

3 Add a spiky four-pointed palm tree leaf at the top of the right-hand dot using a lime green nail art pen or small detail brush dipped in lime green polish.

4 Add another four-pointed leaf to the left of the dots.

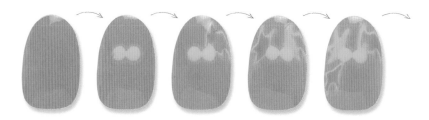

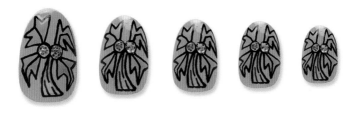

5 Paint a spiky three-pointed palm leaf below the left-hand side of the dots and another three-pointed leaf below the right-hand side of the dots.

6 Using the light metallic orange polish and a small detail brush, paint a curved trunk from beneath the two dots, making it thicker at the cuticle end of the nail.

7 Outline the whole palm with a black nail art pen or small detail brush dipped in black polish; the two dots first, then the leaves and the trunk. Add a line in the centre of each leaf and small vertical lines following the shape of the trunk.

8 Add gold glitter to the two gold dots using a dotting tool. When dry, apply a top coat.

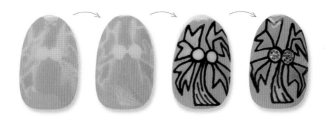

CORAL REEF

Even if you can't take a snorkeling trip to the Maldives, these beautiful coral designs will make you feel as if you were there!

YOU WILL NEED:

nail art pens or polish in bright orange, white and black, fine detail brush (if not using pens), plus base coat and top coat.

1   After prepping the nails and applying a base coat, paint two coats of bright orange polish to all 10 nails. Leave to dry.

2   Using a white nail art pen or small detail brush dipped in white nail polish, draw a shell-like shape by painting an upside-down fan-shaped triangle and filling it in with white.

3   At the point of the shell, paint two small white triangles on either side.

4   Draw more shell-like shapes over the nails, making sure to leave enough room between them to draw the coral shapes.

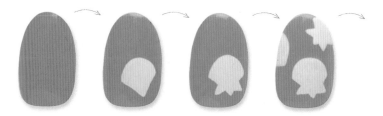

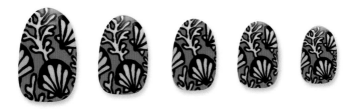

5   Add wavy tree-like patterns behind the shells to create a coral reef effect.

6   When the white is dry, you can start outlining the shapes. Using a black nail art pen or small detail brush dipped in black, outline the shell fan shape, the smaller triangles and the coral reef.

7   Add four lines inside the shell from the top to the point of the triangle, which should divide the shell into five segments. Repeat on all the shells.

8   At the curved top of the shell, draw on a black scalloped edge and fill it in.

9   Leave to dry, then apply a top coat.

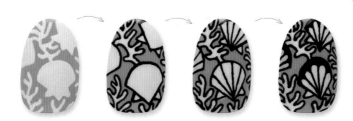

ICE-CREAM CONE

Perfect for a sunny seaside holiday, these cute ice-cream cones look good enough to eat!

YOU WILL NEED:

nail art pens or polish colours in pastel blue, white, pink, black and metallic light orange, fine detail brush (if not using pens), plus base coat and top coat.

1 After prepping and applying a base coat, paint all 10 nails with two coats of pastel blue nail polish. Leave to dry.

2 Using a small detail brush dipped in metallic light orange nail polish, paint a cone shape at the base of the nail.

3 Using a white nail art pen or small detail brush dipped in white polish, draw an ice-cream shape on top of the cone. To do this, draw a fluffy cloud-like shape first and then add an elongated "whip" to a point at the top.

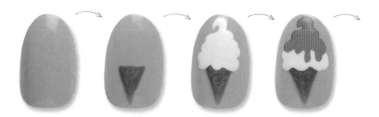

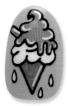

4   Add pink drippy sauce to the top of the ice cream using a pink nail art pen or small detail brush dipped in pink polish.

5   Add a chocolate flake using the same metallic light orange as the cone, and draw small white drips at the bottom of the cone in the blue space.

6   Outline the pink sauce and ice cream with a black nail art pen or small detail brush dipped in black polish.

7   Outline the cone, the flake and the drips in black and add white detailing to the side of the cone and edges of the pink using a white nail art pen or small detail brush.

8   When dry, finish with a top coat to seal.

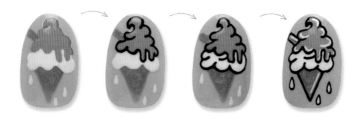

KISS ME QUICK

These red lips are the perfect hint for a Valentine's kiss.

YOU WILL NEED:

nail art pens or polish colours in white, red and black, red glitter nail polish, fine detail brush (if not using pens), plus base coat and top coat.

1   After prepping the nails and applying a base coat, paint all 10 nails with two coats of white nail polish. Leave to dry.

2   Using a red nail art pen or small detail brush dipped in red polish, draw an outline of lips in the centre of the nail.

3   Fill the lips in with red glitter nail polish using a small detail brush.

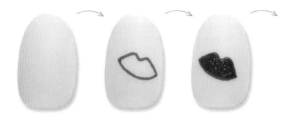

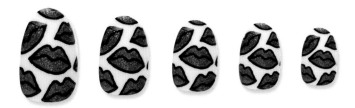

4 Add more lip shapes all over the nail at different angles to create a repeat lip pattern.

5 Outline the lips using a black nail art pen or small detail brush dipped in black polish.

6 Draw a curved black line through each lip shape with a black nail art pen or small detail brush dipped in black polish.

7 Leave to dry, then apply a top coat.

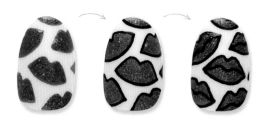

HALLOWEEN COFFINS & PUMPKINS

These two spooky designs will get you in the Halloween spirit!

YOU WILL NEED:

nail art pens or polish colours in black, neon orange and white, fine detail brush (if not using pens), plus base coat and top coat.

Coffins

1 Prep and apply a base coat. Paint six nails with two coats of black nail polish, leaving two feature nails and both thumbs for the neon orange. Leave to dry.

2 Draw a coffin shape, line by line as shown below, in the centre of each nail with a white nail art pen or detail brush dipped in white nail polish.

3 Draw short white lines from four corners of the coffin and join up to complete a 3D coffin shape.

4 Draw more coffins to complete a repeat pattern all over the nail. Add a small white cross at the head of each coffin. When dry, apply a top coat.

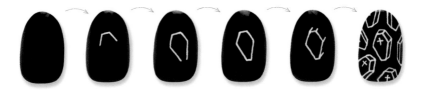

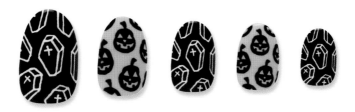

Pumpkins

1   Paint the ring fingers and thumbs with two coats of neon orange polish. Leave to dry.

2   Using a black nail art pen or detail brush dipped in black nail polish, draw the outline of a pumpkin shape towards the top of the nail.

3   Draw two triangles at the top of the pumpkin shape. Draw a small circle below and between the triangles and a line beneath the circle from end to end.

4   Colour the pumpkin shape black, leaving the triangles, circle and mouth shape orange. Draw a little stalk shape at the top of the pumpkin. Add three black teeth – one at the top and two on the bottom – inside the mouth

5   Add more pumpkins to make a repeat pattern all over the nail. When dry, apply a top coat.

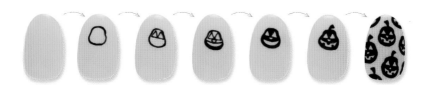

PARISIAN CHIC

Take a trip to the City of Love with this heart design and top it off with an Eiffel Tower!

YOU WILL NEED:

nail art pens or polish in white, red, blue, gold glitter and cornflower blue, fine detail brush (if not using pens), plus base coat and top coat.

I Heart Paris

1   After prepping the nails and applying a base coat, paint six nails (or four, if using the Eiffel Tower option) with two coats of white nail polish. Leave to dry.

2   Draw a big slanted heart outline with a red nail art pen or fine detail brush dipped in red polish. Fill in.

3   Outline the heart with a gold glitter nail art pen or small detail brush dipped in gold glitter polish.

4   Inside the heart write "PARIS" with a white nail art pen or small detail brush dipped in white polish. When dry, add a top coat.

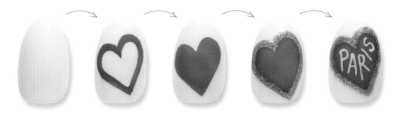

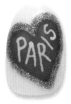

Oui Paris

1 After prepping the nails and applying a base coat, paint the remaining four nails in cornflour blue nail polish. Leave to dry.

2 Using a white nail art pen or small detail brush dipped in white polish, write "bonjour" in curly lettering on a slant across the nail.

3 Add "oui" above "bonjour", slanted in the other direction.

4 Add more French words like "merci", "j'adore", etc., in the same handwriting until the whole nail is covered in words.

5 When the writing is dry, finish with a top coat.

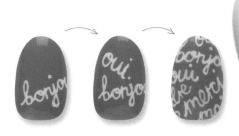

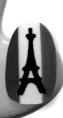

OPTION
For a feature nail, draw an Eiffel Tower in black on a field of red, white and blue stripes, as shown here.

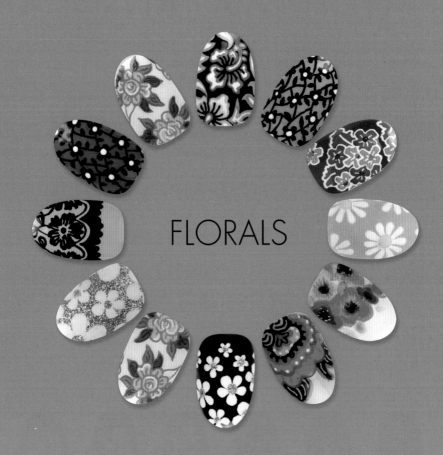

FLORALS

HAWAIIAN

*These exotic blooms will transport you
to a tropical Paradise!*

YOU WILL NEED:

*nail art pens or polish in black, white, yellow, pink, orange and green, dotting tool and
fine detail brush (if not using pens), plus base coat and top coat.*

1   After prepping the nails and applying a base coat, paint all 10 nails with
    two thin coats of black nail polish. Leave to dry.

2   Using a white nail art pen or small detail brush dipped in white nail polish,
    paint a stem shape in the middle of the nail.

3   Using a yellow nail art pen or dotting tool dipped in yellow polish, apply four
    dots of yellow to the top of the white stem shape.

4   Draw a white petal shape next to the stem. Draw your petal with a scalloped
    edge and two lines cutting through to the centre.

5   Draw another white petal directly under the one you have just drawn.

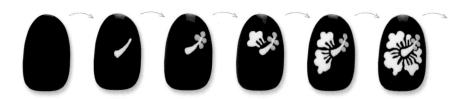

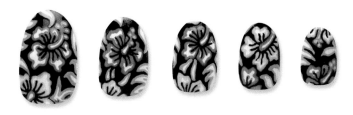

6 Add two more petals around the stem.

7 At the base of the nail, paint the top part of another flower. At the tip, paint white tropical leaf shapes. Add more tropical leaf shapes around the flowers.

8 Outline the stem and yellow dots with an orange nail art pen or small detail brush dipped in orange polish.

9 Outline the flowers, one with pink polish and one with yellow, using nail art pens or a small detail brush dipped in polish.

10 Outline the leaves with green polish, using a green nail art pen or small detail brush dipped in green polish.

11 When dry, apply a top coat to seal.

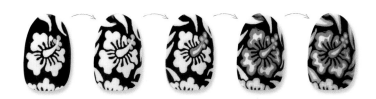

DITSY

This pretty floral design could be the perfect finishing touch to a spring outfit.

YOU WILL NEED:

nail art pens or polish in green, black and white, dotting tool and fine detail brush (if not using pens), plus base coat and top coat.

1 After prepping the nails and applying a base coat, paint each nail with two coats of green polish. Leave to dry.

2 Using a black nail art pen or dotting tool dipped in black polish, apply dots randomly over the nail, leaving enough green space around each one to fit in the rest of the design.

3 Turn the dots you've made into little flowers by adding three or four black dots around each centre dot using the pen or dotting tool.

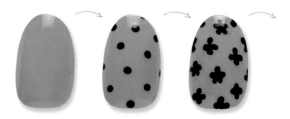

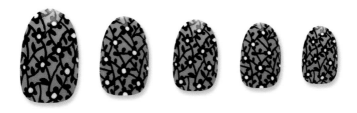

4   In the spaces between the "flowers", paint black lines to make branches connecting the flowers, crossing over each other like a tangled vine design.

5   Draw tiny little leaves on some of the branches.

6   Using a white nail art pen or a dotting tool dipped in white polish, add a dot to the centre of each flower.

7   When dry, finish with a top coat.

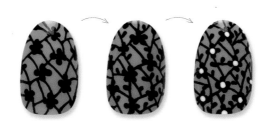

APPLE BLOSSOM

*Create a cluster of blossoms for
a garden-party theme.*

YOU WILL NEED:

*nail art pens or polish in bright blue, pink, red, green and white, fine detail brush
and dotting tool (if not using pens), plus base coat and top coat.*

1   After prepping the nails and applying a base coat, paint all 10 nails with bright
    blue polish. Leave to dry.

2   Using a pink nail art pen or small detail brush dipped in pink polish, draw on
    clusters of flower-like shapes with five petals. Don't completely cover the
    nail – make sure to leave space for the other flowers and leaves. You want to
    have some blue peeking through, too.

3   Next to the pink flowers, paint red flowers clustered together using a red
    nail art pen or small detail brush dipped in red polish. Make some flowers fall
    from the cluster into the blue, but still leaving some blue space visible.

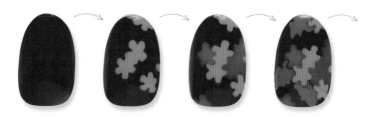

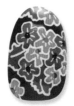

4 On the outer edges of the flower cluster, paint two curly leaf shapes using a green nail art pen or small detail brush dipped in green polish. Paint another curly leaf at the tip of the nail.

5 Outline the pink flowers with a white nail art pen or detail brush dipped in white polish. Then outline the red flowers in white.

6 Outline the green curly leaves in white and add a line down the centre of each leaf.

7 Inside each pink flower, add a dot of green using a nail art pen or a dotting tool dipped in green polish. Add a dot of blue to the centre of each red flower. Paint four dashes of white around each dot for detail.

8 When dry, finish with a top coat to seal.

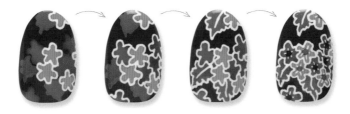

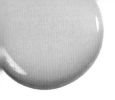

HAZY DAISY

Sweet and innocent, these daisies make a charming, girly design.

YOU WILL NEED:

nail art pens or polish colours in warm grey, white and yellow, dotting tool and fine detail brush (if not using pens), plus base coat and top coat.

1   After prepping the nails and applying a base coat, paint all 10 nails with two coats of warm grey polish. Leave to dry.

2   Using a white nail art pen or a dotting tool dipped in white polish, apply a large dot to the centre top of the nail.

3   Now draw a petal shape at the top of the white dot.

4   Paint on two more petals either side of the first, leaving a small gap between the petals.

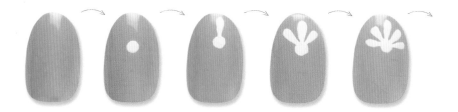

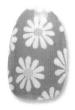

---

5 Paint on two more petals either side of these so you have now have five in total.

6 Add five more petals so you have 10 in total.

7 Repeat steps 2 to 6 to add more daisies and half-daisies, scattered in the remaining grey space.

8 Using a yellow nail art pen or a dotting tool dipped in yellow polish, apply a large dot of yellow to the centre of each daisy.

9 Leave to dry and apply a top coat to seal.

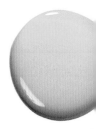

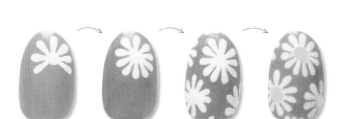

WATERCOLOUR

Eye-popping colours are gently blended to make this super-bright display.

YOU WILL NEED:

nail polish colours in white, bright purple, dark purple, black, yellow, green and various shades of orange, pink and red, aluminium foil or mixing palette, nail polish remover, fine detail brush, plus base coat and top coat.

I Prep the nails and apply a base coat. Paint all 10 nails with two coats of white polish. Then paint a coat of top coat over the white. This is so the white polish is not removed or mixed when you create the watercolour flowers. Leave to dry.

2 Dip a small brush into nail polish remover and mix with some bright purple polish on a piece of aluminium foil or the palette. Paint the purple onto the nail in a flower shape. Add more paint or polish remover to the brush and mix it on the nail to give the flower a washed-out watercolour effect.

3 Mix the darker purple polish with the nail polish remover. Paint it into the centre of the lighter purple and let the colours bleed into each other. You can add more polish or remover and drag the colours into each other to blend.

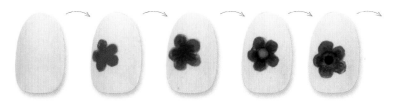

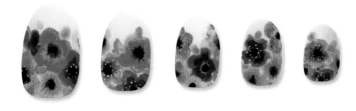

---

4 Mix a little orange polish with nail polish remover and circle into the centre of the flower. Drag the colour into the purple a little. Add a black dot in the centre.

5 Paint a yellow flower next to the purple one. Repeat steps 2 to 4 but use different shades of orange and a hint of purple near the black dot.

6 Create another flower in the same way, this time using pink polishes with a little bit of purple and a black dot in the centre.

7 Create more flowers, this time using reds, oranges and a little bit of purple around the black dot. Add more coloured flowers near the cuticle end of the nail.

8 Mix the bright green polish with a little nail polish remover and paint tiny leaves between the flowers.

9 Add tiny white dots or dashes around the black on a few of the flowers to give detail. When dry, apply a top coat to seal.

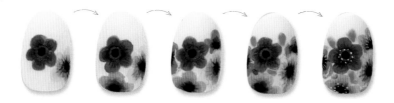

ANKARA

African floral prints, like this one, are some of my favourites. Take a look yourself and see if they can inspire your own nail art designs.

YOU WILL NEED:

nail art pens or polish in yellow, light green, black, lilac, pink, red, dark green and dark purple, fine detail brush (if not using pens), plus base coat and top coat.

1 After prepping the nails and applying a base coat, paint all 10 nails with two coats of yellow polish. Leave to dry.

2 Using a light green nail art pen or small detail brush dipped in light green polish, draw a small "onion"-like shape on each nail with two ovals below it.

3 Using a black nail art pen or small detail brush dipped in black polish, outline the top of the "onion" shape and then add a frill of dots to the outline.

4 Outline the black with lilac, following the frill-like shape. Outline the shape all around with a thick band of pink with a scalloped edge at the top.

5 Using a red nail art pen or brush dipped in red polish, outline the scalloped edge. Draw another, tighter frilled red line halfway through the pink frill.

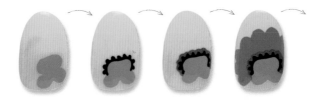

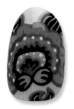

6 Using a dark green nail art pen or brush dipped in dark green polish, draw a line around the light green "onion" shape and an outline around the two light green ovals. Add two curved lines inside each light green oval. Add dark green leaf shapes above the flower, in the yellow space.

7 Outline the leaves in lilac and add lilac line details to the pink frill above the middle red outline. Add a lilac club-like shape to the light green "onion".

8 Paint a dark purple section within the lilac club shape.

9 Using a white nail art pen or a dotting tool dipped in white polish, add dot detailing above the club shape and in the pink frill.

10 Add light green stripe detailing inside the leaves and three pink lines inside the purple club shape.

11 When dry, finish with a top coat to seal.

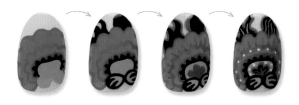

DAISY CHAIN

Make peace not war with this
1960s hippie-inspired design.

YOU WILL NEED:

nail polish colours in black, white and gold glitter, dotting tool, plus base coat and top coat.

1 After prepping the nails and applying a base coat, paint all 10 nails with two coats of black polish. Leave to dry.

2 Using a dotting tool dipped in white polish, place a dot about one-quarter of the way down from the tip of the nail.

3 Above this dot, place another white dot using the dotting tool. This is the first petal of the flower.

4 Place another dot on each side of the first dot, so you now have three petals around the centre dot.

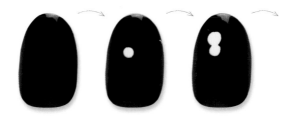

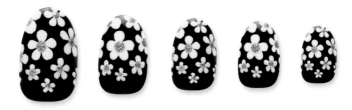

5 Add two more dots below the central one to complete the five-petal flower.

6 Using the same technique, add more flowers around the tip area of the nail. As you get closer to the cuticle end, make the flowers smaller to create a scattered gradient effect. Leave the black space at the cuticle end free of flowers.

7 Using a dotting tool dipped in gold glitter polish, add a dot to the centre of each flower.

8 When dry, finish with a top coat to seal.

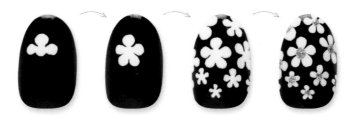

TEACUP ROSES

Decorate your nails for summer with this pretty pink floribunda design.

YOU WILL NEED:

nail art pens or polish in white, pale pink, light green, dark green and dark pink, dotting tool and fine detail brush (if not using pens), plus base coat and top coat.

1   After prepping the nails and applying a base coat, paint all 10 nails with two coats of white polish. Leave to dry.

2   Using a pale pink nail art pen or a dotting tool dipped in pale pink polish, draw a small circle in the middle of the nail. Add a smaller circle to the top of the first pink circle and another pink circle to the left to create petals.

3   Draw another petal to the right of the top petal, but make it slightly curved. To do this, place a dot directly next to another dot, like a figure of eight attached to the central dot. Repeat to create another curved petal opposite.

4   Paint a further two single petals at the bottom to complete the rose shape.

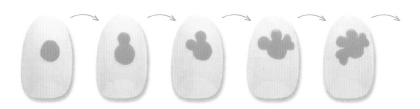

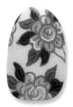

5 Using a light green nail art pen or a small detail brush dipped in light green polish, paint four leaves around the rose shape. Paint four darker green leaves between the light green ones.

6 At the cuticle end, add a half-rose with leaves to make the design look like a repeat pattern across the whole nail.

7 Using a dark pink nail art pen or a brush dipped in dark pink polish, outline the whole rose and the individual petals. Outline the green leaves and add a stem.

8 Add dark pink detail lines within the flower – one or two lines in each petal and two "C" shapes inside each other in the rose's centre. Add a dark pink line detail in each leaf.

9 Paint white shading on the petals and in the rose's centre. When the design is complete and dry on all 10 nails, finish with a top coat.

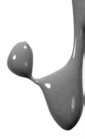

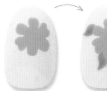   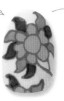 

FLOWER POWER

Paint white stylized flowers on top of a glitter base for a 1960s look.

YOU WILL NEED:

nail art pens or polish in gold glitter and white, fine detail brush and dotting tool (if not using pens), plus base coat and top coat.

1   After prepping the nails and applying a base coat, paint all 10 nails with two coats of gold glitter polish. Leave to dry.

2   Add a small outline of a circle in the centre of the nail using a white nail art pen or a small detail brush dipped in white polish.

3   At the top of the circle, paint a filled-in white dot. This is the first petal of the flower.

4   Add a dot on each side of this first dot so you have three petals around the central circle. Make sure you have a slight gap between petals.

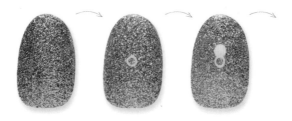

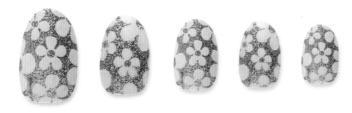

5 Complete the flower by adding two more white dots around the circle to make a five-petal flower.

6 On the right-hand side of the nail, use the same technique to paint flowers in various sizes next to each other.

7 Keep adding flowers using the same dotting technique until the whole nail is covered with the flower pattern.

8 Leave to dry, then apply a top coat to seal.

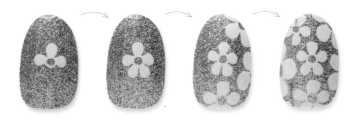

CORAL LACE FLOWERS

This intricate lace design incorporates
fringing and flowers for pretty summer nails.

YOU WILL NEED:

nail art pens or polish in coral and black, fine detail brush (if not using pens),
plus base coat and top coat.

1   After prepping the nails and applying a base coat, paint all 10 nails with
    two coats of coral-coloured polish. Leave to dry.

2   Using a black nail art pen or a dotting tool dipped in black polish, apply
    a black dot about one-quarter of the way from the tip.

3   Draw two petals above the black dot. To do this, draw a scalloped edge
    with three black lines towards the black central dot.

4   Paint another black petal directly below the central dot in the same way
    and add two more petals in the spaces left around the dot.

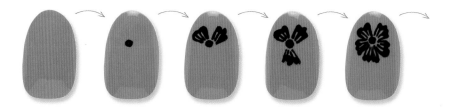

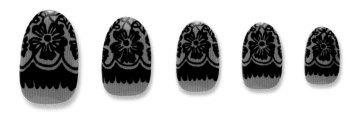

5   Draw a black curved line around the bottom petal and then two curved lines on either side towards the side of the nail. Outline the curved line.

6   Approximately one-quarter above the cuticle end of the nail, draw a black frilly line. Fill in the section from the frill to the curved line to create the fringe.

7   Add a flower on each side of the central flower. You won't fit a whole flower in, so just paint the petals so the design looks like a continuous repeat pattern across the whole nail.

8   At the tip, create some lace detailing by adding lines and swirls.

9   When dry, finish with a top coat.

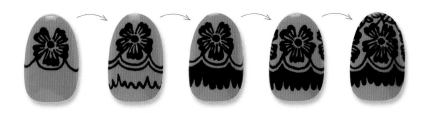

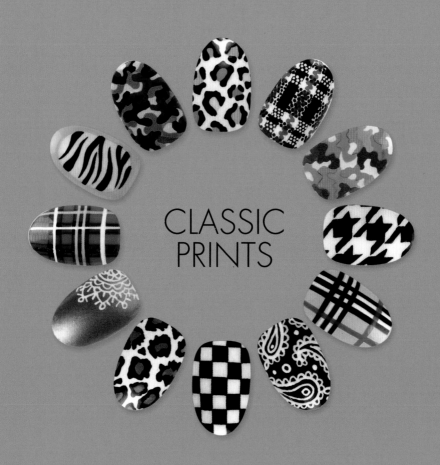

CLASSIC
PRINTS

COLOURFUL
LEOPARD PRINT

*This is a more fun and colourful version
of the classic leopard print.*

YOU WILL NEED:

*nail art pens or polish colours in white, yellow, pink, neon green, neon orange, bright
blue and black, fine detail brush (if not using pens), plus base coat and top coat.*

1   After prepping the nails and applying a base coat, paint two coats of white
    polish on all 10 nails. Leave to dry.

2   Using the bright yellow polish and a detail brush, paint two or three uneven
    yellow spots randomly on each nail. If you prefer, use the brush from the
    polish bottle.

3   Next paint two or three neon pink spots on each nail.

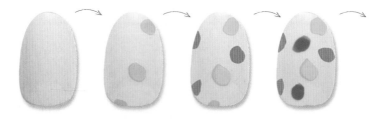

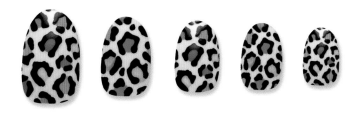

4   Repeat with neon green, orange and bright blue polish colours to create different-coloured spots, making sure you leave enough gaps between them to add black outlines.

5   Using a black nail art pen or a detail brush dipped in black polish, paint "C"-shaped lines around the coloured spots to create the leopard-print motif.

6   Add three black dashes between the coloured spots.

7   When dry, seal with a top coat.

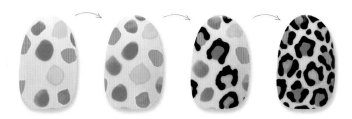

LAUNDRY BAG

A great variation on a checked pattern, this design captures the woven texture of a laundry bag.

YOU WILL NEED:

nail art pens or polish colours in white, navy blue and red, striping brush and fine detail brush (if not using pens), plus base coat and top coat.

1   After prepping the nails and applying a base coat, apply two coats of white nail polish to all 10 nails. Leave to dry.

2   Paint a thick vertical line at the left-hand side of the nail using a striping brush dipped in navy blue polish.

3   Paint another thick navy blue line on the right-hand side of the nail so you now have two thick blue lines with a large vertical band of white running down the middle of the nail.

4   Widthways across the centre of the nail, paint a line of tiny navy dots using a navy blue nail art pen or a small detail brush dipped in navy polish.

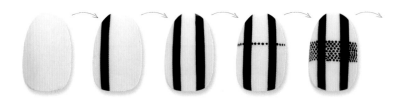

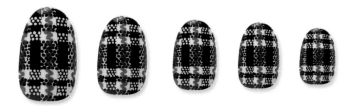

5 Continue painting on rows of dots in navy blue in a band across the nail. Paint about nine rows in total.

6 Leaving a gap on either side of the band of dots, paint two rows of dots at the top and bottom. Leaving a gap between these lines, add rows of dots at the tip and cuticle end of the nail.

7 In the sections between the rows of dots, within the two thick navy stripes, paint white dots with a white nail art pen or small detail brush dipped in white polish.

8 Using a red nail art pen or a small detail brush dipped in red polish, draw a zig-zag line of dots down the centre of the nail. Draw two more zig-zag lines on the left- and right-hand sides.

9 When dry, finish with a top coat.

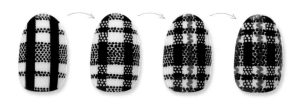

CAMOUFLAGE

A utility-chic fashion favourite, this camo is an urban take on the army print.

YOU WILL NEED:

nail art pens or polish colours in light olive green, dark green, reddish brown and dark brown, fine detail brush (if not using pens), plus base coat and top coat.

I   After prepping the nails and applying a base coat, paint all 10 nails with light olive green nail polish. Leave to dry.

2   Using a nail-art pen or small detail brush dipped in dark green polish, draw on irregular freeform shapes on the nail.

3   Add some more dark green "camo" shapes in the olive green space. Make sure you leave enough space to add two more colours of shapes.

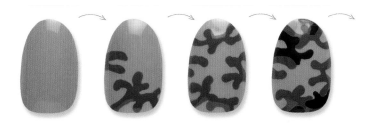

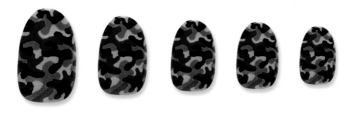

4   Add more irregular "camo" shapes, this time using reddish/brown nail art pen or polish and a small detail brush.

5   Add more reddish/brown irregular "camo" shapes to the nail. You can fit them between the dark green shapes or place them on top. Just make sure you leave some space for the last colour shapes and that you have some olive green visible in the finished design.

6   Using the dark brown polish and a small detail brush, or a nail art pen, paint the final "camo" print shapes between and on top of some of the existing shapes, leaving some olive green visible. When dry, apply a top coat.

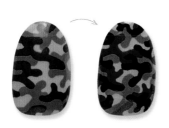

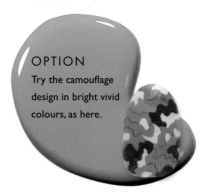

OPTION
Try the camouflage design in bright vivid colours, as here.

HOUNDSTOOTH

Classy and traditional, this duotone weave pattern is based on broken check shapes.

YOU WILL NEED:

nail art pens or polish colours in white and black, fine detail brush (if not using pens), plus base coat and top coat.

1   After prepping and applying a base coat, paint all 10 nails with two coats of white nail polish. Leave to dry.

2   Just above the centre of the nail, draw a small black square using a black nail art pen or small detail brush dipped in black polish.

3   Paint a short diagonal black line from the bottom left corner of the square.

4   Paint another short diagonal black line from the top right corner of the square.

5   Paint a small black triangle shape at the top of the left-hand corner of the square.

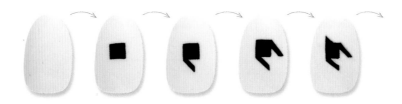

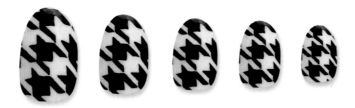

6   Add another small black triangle shape to the left-hand side of the square, perpendicular to the first triangle. This now completes the basis of the houndstooth pattern.

7   Repeat steps 2 to 6 directly beneath the first houndstooth, with the top right corner of the square meeting the left "leg" of the first houndstooth.

8   Paint another houndstooth directly above the first, with the "leg" of the houndstooth meeting the top right corner of the first houndstooth.

9   Fill both sides of the nail with the black houndstooth design, fitting the houndsteeth next to each other so you create a white houndstooth between the black ones.

10 When all 10 nails are complete and dry, finish with a top coat.

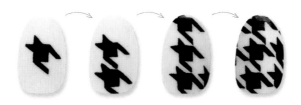

PINK HERITAGE PRINT

For a variation, try this Burberry-inspired pattern in the classic tan, black, white and red.

YOU WILL NEED:

nail polish colours in pastel pink, white, black and red, striping brush, plus base coat and top coat.

1   After prepping and applying a base coat, paint all 10 nails with two coats of pastel pink nail polish. Leave to dry.

2   Using a striping brush and white polish, paint a thick white band at the left-hand side of the nail, leaving a gap of pink at the side.

3   Paint a white band across the middle of the nail so you have something that looks like an off-centre cross.

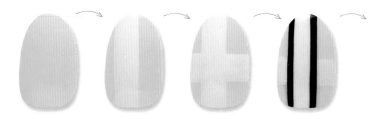

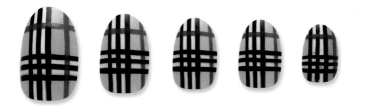

4 Outline the vertical white band with two stripes using a striping brush dipped in black polish.

5 Outline the horizontal white band with two black stripes in the same way.

6 Add a black line in the middle of both the vertical and horizontal white bands.

7 Using a striping brush dipped in red polish, paint a vertical red stripe on the right-hand side of the nail.

8 Add a horizontal red stripe at the tip of the nail.

9 When all 10 nails are complete and dry, finish with a top coat.

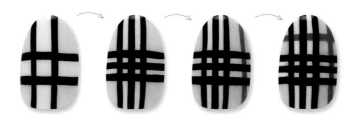

PAISLEY BANDANA

The paisley design is easier to do when limited to just two colours but you could add more colours to the mix for a brighter effect.

YOU WILL NEED:

nail art pens or polish in black and white, fine detail brush (if not using pens), plus base coat and top coat.

1   After prepping the nails and applying a base coat, paint all 10 nails with two coats of black polish. Leave to dry.

2   Using a white nail art pen or small detail brush dipped in white polish, draw a small outlined white circle centred about one-quarter of the way from the tip.

3   Using a white nail art pen or detail brush dipped in white polish, draw a "kidney" shape with a pointed end around the small circle.

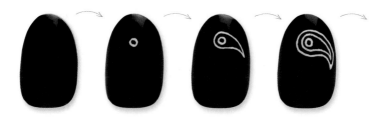

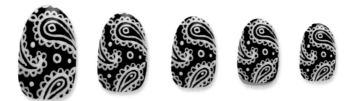

4   Outline the kidney shape with another white line.

5   Draw a frilly edge all the way around the second kidney outline.
    Add a small "lemon" shape outline to the top of the frill.

6   Draw another paisley shape below the first.

7   Draw on more paisley shapes in the rest of the black space on the nail
    for a repeat paisley pattern.

8   In the black spaces between the paisley shapes, draw little circle outlines.

9   Leave to dry, then finish with a top coat.

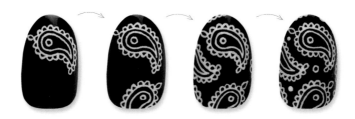

CHECKERBOARD

Check? Checkmate? You'll always be winning with this classic monochrome design!

YOU WILL NEED:

nail polish colours in black and white, striping brush, plus base coat and top coat.

1   After prepping the nails and applying a base coat, paint all 10 nails with two coats of white nail polish. Leave to dry.

2   Using a striping brush dipped in black polish, paint two vertical lines down the centre of the nail with a 1mm (1/32 inch) gap between them.

3   Paint more vertical black stripes down the nail at 1mm (1/32 inch) intervals.

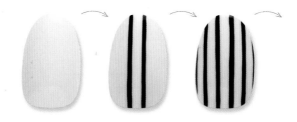

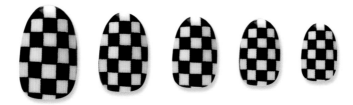

4 Paint two black stripes horizontally across the centre of the nail at 1mm (⅟₃₂ inch) intervals.

5 Continue painting horizontal black stripes until the nail is covered with a grid-like pattern.

6 Using a small detail brush dipped in black polish, paint black in each alternating square to create a checkerboard design. Repeat on all 10 nails.

7 When dry, finish with a top coat.

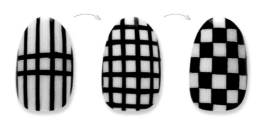

SNOW LEOPARD

*Evocative of snowscapes and frozen tundra,
this animal print will become a winter favourite.*

YOU WILL NEED:

nail art pens or polish colours in white, grey and black, fine detail brush (if not using pens), plus base coat and top coat.

1 After prepping the nails and applying a base coat, paint all 10 nails with two coats of white nail polish. Leave to dry.

2 Using a detail brush dipped in grey polish, paint an uneven spot of grey in the centre of the nail. If you prefer, use the brush from the polish bottle.

3 Fill the nail with grey spots in varying shapes. The more random the better!

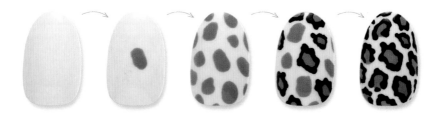

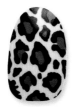

4 Outline each spot with a wobbly black line, using a black nail art pen or a small detail brush dipped in black polish.

5 Outline the rest of the spots with disjointed wobbly black lines looking like "C"-shaped lines and a dash.

6 When all 10 nails are complete and dry, apply a top coat.

TOP TIPS

• *Leopard print looks best when the spots are different shapes and sizes. Don't be too precious as the more random the better – just like the real thing!*

• *If you're just starting to learn how to use nail art pens, leopard print is a great first design to master. The pens give you more freedom than a brush to create curves, like the leopard outlines here.*

LACE PATTERN

Try placing the lace design on different parts of each individual nail for a whole set.

YOU WILL NEED:

nail art pens or polish in oxblood red and white, fine detail brush (if not using pens), plus base coat and top coat.

1   After prepping the nails and applying a base coat, paint all 10 nails with oxblood red nail polish. Leave to dry.

2   Using a white nail art pen or small detail brush dipped in white polish, draw a semi-circle at the cuticle end of the nail, starting from the centre base of the nail to the right-hand side.

3   Leave a small gap and outline with another white semi-circle.

4   Draw a white frill on the second semi-circle. Leave a tiny gap and outline the frill with a second white scalloped line.

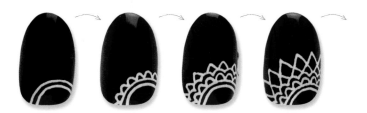

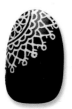

5 Between each scalloped bump, paint a white triangle-shaped outline.

6 Between each triangle, paint a larger white diamond outline shape.

7 Add little white outline circles to the tip of the large diamonds and two dashes of white on either side. Add vertical dashes in the large diamond shapes.

8 Inside the semi-circle at the base of the nail, draw petal-like shapes side by side and finish with a semi-circle line running through them.

9 When dry, apply a top coat.

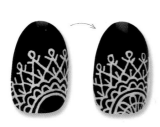

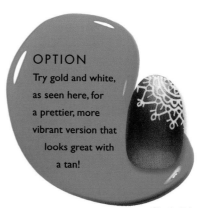

OPTION
Try gold and white, as seen here, for a prettier, more vibrant version that looks great with a tan!

TARTAN

Get Highland style with this traditional Scottish plaid.

YOU WILL NEED:

nail polish colours in red, green, black, metallic navy, white and yellow, striping brush, fine detail brush, plus base coat and top coat.

1   After prepping the nails and applying a base coat, apply two coats of red nail polish to all 10 nails. Leave to dry.

2   Using a striping brush dipped in green polish, paint two thick vertical green stripes about 1mm (1/32 inch) apart. Place them closer to the left-hand side so you have a bigger gap of red on the right-hand side of the nail.

3   Paint two thick green horizontal stripes across the nail. Place them slightly closer to the tip side of the nail so you have a bigger gap at the cuticle end.

4   Using a small detail brush dipped in black polish, paint four little squares in the spaces where the thick green stripes meet.

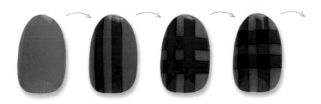

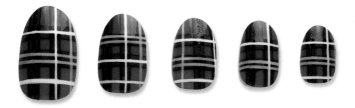

5 Using a striping brush dipped in metallic navy, paint a thin vertical line inside the vertical left-hand green stripe.

6 Using a striping brush dipped in white polish, paint a thin vertical line inside the vertical right-hand green stripe.

7 Using a striping brush dipped in yellow polish, paint two thin horizontal lines inside the top green horizontal stripe. Add a vertical yellow stripe along the right-hand side.

8 Now paint a thin white horizontal line in the lower horizontal green stripe. Add another thin white line parallel at the cuticle end of the nail.

9 When all nails are complete and dry, finish with a top coat.

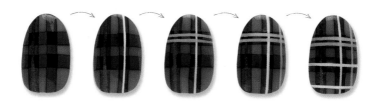

ZEBRA PRINT

Go wild with monochrome zebra stripes! Experiment with other colours, too – a bright neon base with black stripes looks amazing.

YOU WILL NEED:

nail polish colours in white and black, striping brush, plus base coat and top coat.

1 After prepping the nails and applying a base coat, paint all 10 nails with two coats of white polish. Leave to dry.

2 Using a striping brush dipped in black polish, draw a horizontal "Y" shape from the centre left-hand side of the nail. Make the point thinner as you get closer to the right-hand side by applying less pressure with the brush.

3 On the right-hand side of the nail, paint another horizontal "Y" shape above the first "Y" shape, from right to left with the point close to the left-hand side.

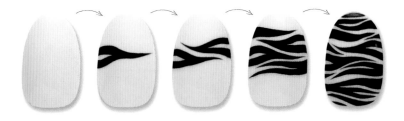

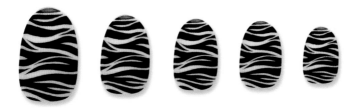

4 Above this, on the left-hand side of the nail, paint a single triangular-shaped zebra stripe.

5 Below the first "Y" shape, paint a forked zebra stripe. To do this, place two curved stripes next to each other.

6 Add more curved and forked stripes from left to right at the tip and cuticle end of the nail. Make sure some stripes go across the whole of the nail.

7 When you have completed all 10 nails and they are dry, finish with a top coat.

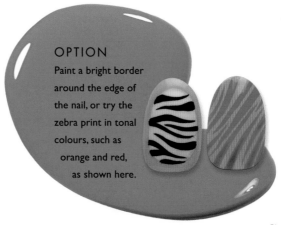

OPTION
Paint a bright border around the edge of the nail, or try the zebra print in tonal colours, such as orange and red, as shown here.

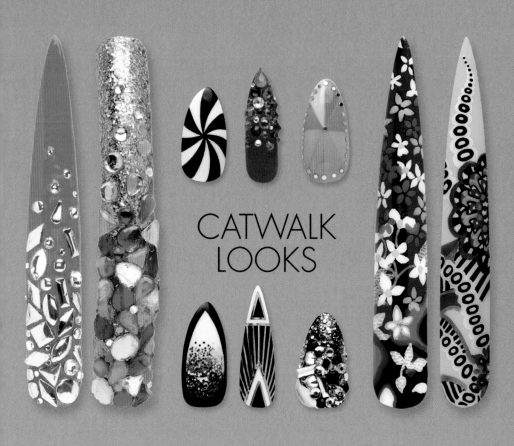

CATWALK
LOOKS

EMBELLISHED OPULENCE

The mix of deep reds and royal blue give this diamond-encrusted nail design an opulent feel.

YOU WILL NEED:

nail polish in royal blue, nail glue, wooden cuticle stick or tweezers, 10 teardrop-shaped red crystals, selection of crystals in varying sizes and shades of red, small clear crystals, 3D red beads, plus base coat and top coat.

1   After prepping the nails and applying a base coat, paint nails with two coats of royal blue nail polish. Leave to dry.

2   Apply a little nail glue to the tip of the nail and, using a wooden cuticle stick or tweezers, place a teardrop-shaped red crystal into the glue and press down lightly. Add a tiny round crystal on either side of the teardrop, one red and one clear, then a large round red crystal below the smaller red one.

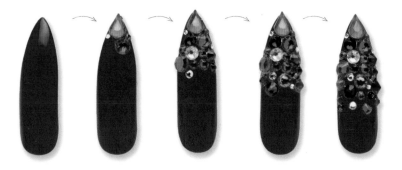

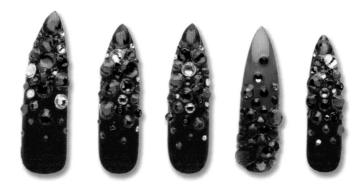

3 Keep applying more nail glue and placing more crystals close together in rows down the nail. Use varying sizes of round crystals in different shades of red, interspersed with clear crystals.

4 Keep applying glue and now intersperse with smaller crystals and add 3D red beads to the mix.

5 About halfway down the nail, start applying smaller crystals and 3D red beads individually, separating them from the bulk of closely packed crystals.

6 In the remaining blue space, apply individual smaller crystals further apart from each other to create a fade effect. Leave a small section of blue polish clear at the cuticle end of the nail.

7 When the design is dry, apply a top coat.

For the Full Set: Try painting one or two feature nails in a deep red polish and apply blue crystals from the cuticle end instead, scattering them out towards the tip.

'60s SWIRL

This bold monochrome '60s Op Art-inspired design really makes a statement.

YOU WILL NEED:

nail polish colours in white and black, striping brush, plus base coat and top coat.

1   After prepping the nails and applying a base coat, paint all 10 nails with two coats of white nail polish. When dry, place a tiny black dot in the centre of each nail.

2   Using a striping brush and black polish, paint two curved lines starting in the centre of the nail (where you placed the tiny black dot) towards the tip to form a twist/fan shape.

3   Fill in between the lines with black polish, creating a solid curved swirl shape.

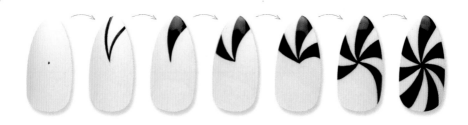

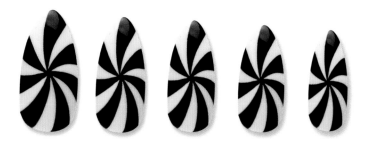

4   Leaving an equal gap, repeat steps 2 and 3 to create a second curved swirl shape to the top left at the tip.

5   Leaving another equal gap, repeat with a third curved swirl shape to the top right of the tip.

6   Repeat with two further swirl shapes to the sides of the nail, remembering to leave equal gaps between.

7   Finish with two final swirl shapes towards the bottom of the cuticle to create the total swirl effect. When dry, apply a top coat.

TOP TIP

• *When you start, place a dot in the centre using black polish to use as your centre guide. You can also place tiny dots on the edge of the nail to guide your curved lines.*

FLOWER GARDEN

This intricate floral set of stiletto nail tips was inspired by the beautiful catwalk prints of fashion designer Peter Pilotto.

YOU WILL NEED:

nail art pens or polish colours in dark blue and metallic blue, lime green, metallic green, white, yellow and orange, striping brush, dotting tool and fine detail brush (if not using pens), plus base and top coats.

1   After prepping the nails and applying a base coat, paint all 10 stiletto nails with dark blue nail polish. When dry, use a striping brush dipped in metallic blue to paint a thick vertical stripe down the centre of the nail.

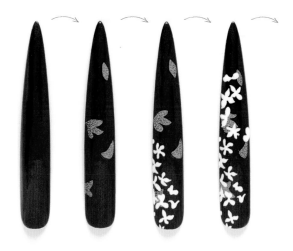

2 Using a lime green nail art pen or a fine detail brush dipped in lime green polish, paint four leaf-like shapes down the nail. When the lime green is dry, use a metallic green nail art pen or brush to paint little squiggles inside each "leaf" shape for added detail.

3 Using a white nail art pen or detail brush dipped in white polish, paint falling flower-like shapes on the left-hand side of the nail. Vary the shape and size.

4 Continue painting falling white flowers at the left-hand side of the nail, leaving a small gap free at the tip. Have some flowers scattered over towards the centre but the flowers should be predominately placed at the left-hand side. Again, vary the shape and size of the flowers.

5 At the tip, paint more scattered flower shapes, but this time keep the flowers smaller and more consistent in size. They should have four pointed petals placed around a central gap. Also place one or two in the gaps at the centre and cuticle end of the nail.

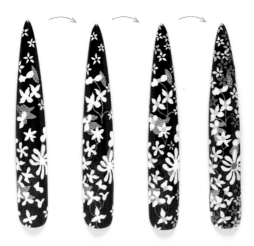

continued...

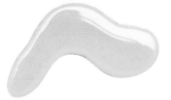

6   Add a much larger daisy-shaped flower about one-quarter of the way up the nail. Make the petals more rounded, curved and elongated, and branching from a white central circle.

7   Using the lime green nail art pen or brush dipped in lime green polish, paint wiggly stems to adjoin some of the flowers on the left-hand side.

8   Using a dotting tool or nail art pen, add dots of yellow to the flower centres, apart from the smaller flowers and the large daisy.

9   Paint on more of the smaller pointed-petal flowers, this time in yellow, scattered at the tip and cuticle ends. Scatter one or two flowers between the other flowers in the centre and right-hand side of the nail, but keep them predominately at the tip and cuticle.

10 Using a dotting tool or nail art pen, paint an orange dot in the centre of the large daisy. In the spaces at the cuticle end and tip, paint more of the smaller shaped pointed-petal flowers, this time in orange. Scatter them between the other flowers and place one or two in the centre at the right-hand side. Leave to dry, then apply a top coat.

Option: For shorter, more wearable nails, recreate smaller sections of the design or paint just a few scattered flowers onto a base of metallic blue.

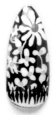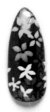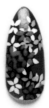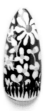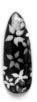

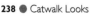

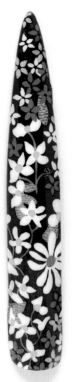
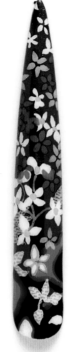
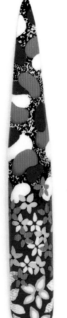
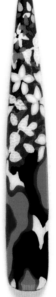
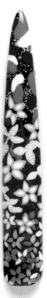
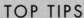

TOP TIPS

• For each flower, start off with a white dot as a central guide for the surrounding petals.

• *This design is quite random and tightly packed, so if you make a mistake you can always just cover it up with more flower shapes.*

GOLDEN RAINBOW

I first created these stand-out rainbow-coloured, gem-encrusted talons for M.I.A.'s album artwork.

YOU WILL NEED:

nail polish in gold glitter, nail glue, wooden cuticle stick, dotting tool or tweezers, crystals in a variety of colours and shapes, small clear crystals, plus base coat and top coat.

1   After prepping the nails and applying a base coat, paint all 10 nails with two coats of gold glitter polish. Leave to dry.

2   Apply a small amount of glue to the cuticle end of the nail. Using a wooden cuticle stick, dotting tool or tweezers, pick up different colours and shapes of crystals and place them along the width of the nail at the cuticle end.

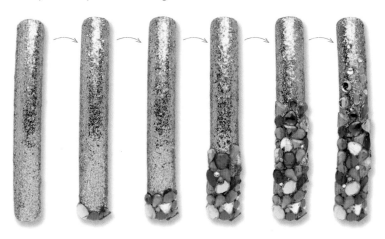

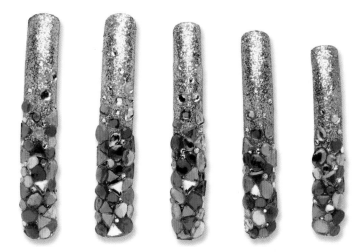

3 Apply more nail glue above the first row and stick on more crystals, ensuring they fit close together with minimal gaps; it's important to do this in stages as the nail glue dries quickly.

4 Apply more crystals in this way for about three-quarters of the length of the nail and then start to add them individually, separating them from the closely packed area to create a scattered effect.

5 Add a few more scattered crystals in the remaining gold space and finish with smaller scattered clear ones to complete the fade. Apply a top coat over the nails for longevity and added shine.

TOP TIP

• *If using acrylic gemstones, be careful not to get nail glue on top of the gems as this can reduce the shine.*

ART DECO SUNBURST

The luxurious Art Deco style of the 1920s inspired this "V"-shaped golden sunburst design.

YOU WILL NEED:

nail polish colours in white and black, striping brush, gold striping tape, tweezers and stork (embroidery) scissors, plus base coat and top coat.

1   After prepping the nails and applying a base coat, paint all 10 nails with two coats of white nail polish. Leave to dry.

2   Using a striping brush, paint a black "V" shape from the cuticle towards the tip, approximately one-third of the way along the length of the nail.

3   Using the striping brush, paint a black horizontal line across the width of the nail, approximately one-third of the way down from the tip of the nail.

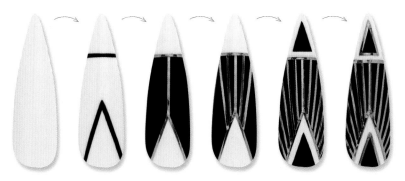

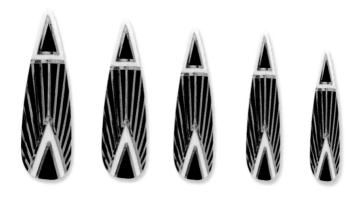

4 Fill in the middle third of the nail with black polish, leaving the tip and cuticle "V" shape white.

5 Using gold striping tape, cut lengths and apply to the "V" shape, along the horizontal width at the top and vertically down the centre of the nail.

6 Now apply two lengths of gold striping tape diagonally on either side of the central tape, leaving a small gap.

7 Continue applying the gold striping tape as for the step 6, but place it so that the gold stripes are wider apart at the top of the nail to create a fan shape. Continue until you have covered the black area of polish.

8 Using the striping brush or a fine detail brush and black nail polish, paint two triangle shapes, one on the cuticle area and one on the nail tip, leaving an even white border on the outside.

9 Apply gold striping tape around both triangle shapes. Finish with a top coat.

DIAMONDS
& STUDS

Let it rain diamonds and studs on these hot pink stilettos! This design can be easily translated into shorter, wearable lengths.

YOU WILL NEED:

nail polish in pink, nail glue, wooden cuticle stick, dotting tool or tweezers, round gold studs in varying sizes, diamond-shaped gold studs, clear crystals in varying shapes and sizes, plus base coat and top coat.

1   After prepping the nails and applying a base coat, paint all 10 nails with two coats of pink nail polish. Leave to dry.

2   Apply a small amount of nail glue to the cuticle end of the nail, and using a wooden cuticle stick, dotting tool or tweezers, apply a large round gold stud to the left-hand side of the cuticle. Sit a large diamond-shaped stud next to this and a smaller round gold stud to the right. Between these gold shapes, apply small clear crystals.

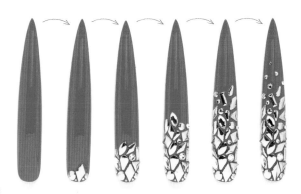

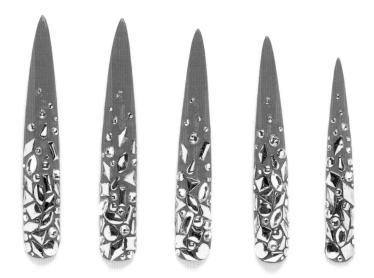

3 Apply more nail glue above this layer of embellishments and place more gold studs in varying shapes interspersed with different shapes of clear crystals. Choose shapes that fit nicely into each other, but leave a tiny gap of pink between each embellishment.

4 Keep applying more nail glue and studs and crystals, leaving tiny gaps of pink between each one, along one-quarter of the nail.

5 Continue in the same way, but start spacing the crystals and studs further apart from each other.

6 Now add some smaller studs and crystals, spaced further apart to create a scattered effect, but leave a small section of pink at the tip clear of any embellishments. Finish with a top coat.

HARLEQUIN

Metallic embellishments contrast nicely with the soft pastel shades in this geometric design, giving an edge to the kaleidoscopic effect.

YOU WILL NEED:

nail polish colours in lilac, pale coral, darker coral, pale blue, pale yellow, purple, green and deep purple, striping brush, wooden cocktail stick, gold flat stones, plus base coat and top coat.

1   After prepping the nails and applying a base coat, paint all 10 nails with lilac nail polish. Leave to dry.

2   Using a striping brush, apply a thin line of pale coral polish vertically down the centre of the nail from cuticle to tip. This will act as your guide for the design.

3   Using the striping brush and the same coral polish, paint one-eighth of the nail to the left side of the centre line at the cuticle end, and do the same with the darker coral colour to the right side at the tip. You can ensure the segments are the same size by matching the line of each segment diagonally across the nail.

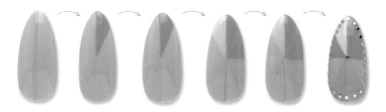

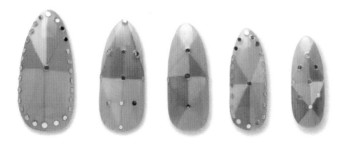

4   Using your striping brush and pale blue polish, paint another one-eighth segment to the left at the bottom at the cuticle end, directly next to and mirroring the light coral one.

5   Using your striping brush and pale yellow polish, paint another one-eighth segment to the left side at the tip end, directly next to and mirroring the darker segment of coral.

6   Using your striping brush and purple polish, paint a one-eighth segment to the top right side of the nail, splitting the area of lilac directly in half.

7   Using your striping brush and green polish, paint a one-eighth segment at the bottom left of the nail, splitting the other area of lilac directly in half.

8   Using your striping brush and deep purple polish, paint a one-eighth segment on the top left side of the nail – the last eighth of the nail shows the original lilac polish. You should now have eight different-coloured segments in total.

9   When dry apply a top coat. While this is still wet, place gold flat stones around the edge of the nail and one in the centre using a cocktail stick.

10 Finish with another layer of top coat to seal in the flat stones.

OUTLINE FADE

This dramatic monochrome design works well on pointed stiletto nails but also looks great on shorter lengths.

YOU WILL NEED:

nail polish colours in white, black, dark metallic grey, silver glitter and fine silver glitter, striping brush, fine detail brush, plus base coat and top coat.

1   After prepping the nails and applying a base coat, paint all 10 nails with white nail polish. Leave to dry.

2   Using a striping brush, apply a thick border of black polish around the entire nail, ensuring you follow the pointed shape of the nail tip.

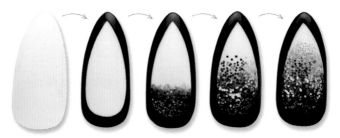

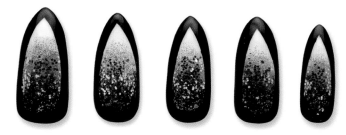

3 Using a fine detail brush, apply the dark metallic grey polish inside the black border to about one-quarter of the way up the nail. Clean your brush and brush the metallic grey into the white as it dries to create a faded effect.

4 On top of the faded metallic grey, apply silver glitter polish and brush towards the tip to create a glitter fade, leaving a small area of the white free.

5 Using very fine glitter polish and a fine detail brush, brush up into the white, leaving a tiny gap of white free at the tip.

6 Leave to dry, then apply a top coat.

TOP TIP

• *For the glitter fade, don't overload your brush. Wherever you want the fade, use less polish on the brush and brush upward. You can go back and build up glitter in the places where you want more of a solid coverage when the design has had a little time to dry.*

INDIAN FLOWERS

The stunning prints of fashion designer Manish Arora were the inspiration behind this beautiful, detailed design.

YOU WILL NEED:

nail art pens or polish colours in white, neon yellow, metallic green, pink, gold, lime green, neon pink, red and black, a fine detail brush or dotting tool (if not using pens), plus base coat and top coat.

1   Prep the nails and apply a base coat. Neon colours always look better and brighter on top of a white base, so paint all 10 nails in white first, leave to dry and then paint two coats of neon yellow nail polish on top. Leave to dry.

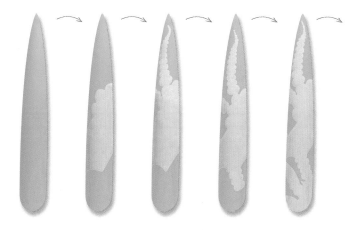

2 Using a white nail art pen or fine detail brush dipped in white polish, draw a white diagonal block section with a curved bottom edge and three curved top edges (as if you were drawing a large flower) in the centre of the nail.

3 On top of the curved-edged "half-flower", paint white ovals sitting on top of each other, varying in size from large to small all the way up towards the tip. Add the start of this oval "stack" at the left side, as if it was falling off the nail.

4 Paint the start of another oval stack extending to about halfway towards the cuticle. This time don't make the ovals go too small; you want to paint about four, all similar in size.

5 Paint the cuticle end with more white polish, and add another oval stack at the left of the nail with a small petal shape between the two stacks. At the left-hand cuticle corner, create a curve. This completes the basic starting shape of the design.

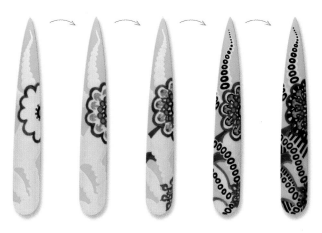

continued...

6 Using a nail art pen or brush, paint a thick outline in metallic green on the "half-flower". There should be six curved edges. Paint a pink half-circle in what would be the centre of the flower. When the pink is dry, outline in metallic green. When the green is dry, add six gold dots around it using a dotting tool.

7 Paint a large gold circle on top of each small gold dot. When dry, paint a smaller green dot in the centre of each large gold circle. Using lime green polish, add a small dot in the centre of the pink circle.

8 Inside each scalloped edge of the flower, paint a gold "mushroom" shape with the "stalks" coming out from the gold circles. To do this, first paint a line from the circle and then paint a crescent moon shape on top.

9 Inside each mushroom shape, paint a smaller mushroom shape in neon pink. Using a red nail art pen or fine detail brush dipped in red polish, draw pointed petal shapes between each mushroom. When the neon pink is dry, add a red triangle detail to the top of each mushroom. Now paint a curved red line underneath the flower towards the left-hand corner of the nail.

10 At the right-hand cuticle end of the nail, on the white base petal shape, draw a small flower. To do this, draw a red half circle with red dots around it. Add gold pointed petal shapes on top and then larger red pointed petal shapes on top of the gold.

11 Using a nail art pen or fine detail brush, outline the mushroom shapes with a thin black line. Inside the white top oval stack, paint black rings scaling from large to a tiny dot at the tip. Draw more rings in the side oval stack and in the one that runs across the nail through the second flower. Also place black rings in the white oval stack next to this.

12 Using a gold polish and a fine detail brush add a thick line next to both red lines and outline the two white curves with a gold band.

13 Using a fine detail brush dipped in black polish, add black wedge-shaped sections to the scalloped edge between the mushroom shapes and the metallic green outline.

14 Using a fine detail brush dipped in black polish, add black diagonal lines to the area under the large flower and vertical black lines under start of the band of rings that runs through the centre of the nail. Add diagonal black lines above the last band of oval rings and diagonal lines in the opposite direction in the left-hand side, near the cuticle. When the design is dry, finish with a top coat.

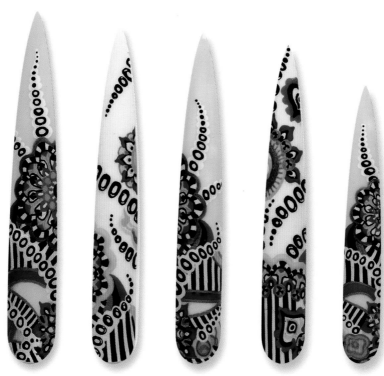

DIAMONDS IN THE ROUGH

It's all about sparkle and texture in this geologically inspired design.
Use all sorts of shapes and sizes of embellishments to build up the effect.

YOU WILL NEED:

nail polish in metallic grey glitter, nail glue, wooden cuticle stick or tweezers, variety of nail art embellishments including leaf-shaped gold studs, black crystals in varying sizes, clear marquise-shaped crystals, 3D pear-shaped gold crystals, gold foil pieces, baguette-shaped gold studs, sequins, aurora borealis crystals, gold flat stones and beads, plus base coat and top coat.

1   After prepping the nails and applying a base coat, paint all 10 nails with metallic grey glitter nail polish. Leave to dry.

2   Place a small amount of nail glue on the right-hand side of the cuticle end of the nail. Using tweezers or a cuticle stick, stick on a leaf-shaped gold stud.

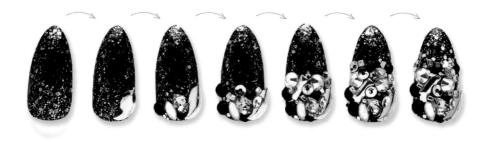

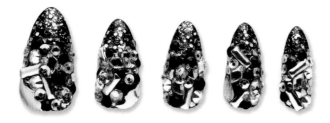

3   Apply more glue along the cuticle end and add a small black crystal, then a clear marquise-shaped crystal, and then a slightly larger black crystal in a line.

4   Using more nail glue, apply a 3D pear-shaped gold crystal above the black crystal, placed next to the leaf stud.

5   Apply more nail glue above the embellishments and add a line of black crystals, gold foil pieces, gold sequins and gold beads, all tightly fitted together.

6   Add more nail glue and continue adding embellishments, including baguette-shaped gold studs and aurora borealis crystals, mixed in with smaller round gold-coloured crystals as well as more sequins and beads.

7   Continue applying nail glue and a mixture of all the embellishments, packing them close together and placing some on top of each other for a 3D effect. Leave about a third of the metallic grey still visible at the tip.

8   Apply a little more nail glue or top coat to the tip and stick small gold flat stones around the top of the embellishments. Place more gold flat stones at the tip, dotted around for a fade effect. Finish with a top coat.

AUTHOR ACKNOWLEDGEMENTS

A huge thank you to the following for all their help, contribution and support with this book and for their continued support in my career:

Catherine Greenslade, Joseph Harris, Katy Harris-Greenslade, David Greenslade, Tristan Harper, Lucy Cole

Also, Emma Davies, Niki Byrne at OPI UK, Shikira Austin, Levanah Reyes-Wainwright & Amy Betsworth at Coty, the whole team at OPI USA: Suzi, Ruthi, Brenda, Lauren, Jaqueleen, Elsa, Gavrielle, Eric, Vu and Robert Nguyen (Mr. Nail Art), Caroline Dawe & Beth Thomas at Barry M, Leanne McIntosh at Original Additions, Sim Stevens at Sparkle, Frances Rickard at Mac, everyone at Beauty Seen – Nisha Smith, Charlie Ross and Jodie Edwards, Michael Robbins at Zwilling J.A. Henckels, Alex Fox, Helena Biggs and Kayleigh Baker at *Scratch* magazine.

Thank you to the following brands for supplying product for the book:

OPI, Coty, Barry M, Elegant Touch, Nailene, Alessandro, Tweezerman, Revlon, Topshop Beauty, MAC, The New Black, Dior, Mr. Nail Art, Madam Glam, Nail HQ.

THE ILLUSTRATED NAIL

Find more nail art designs on my website, Instagram and Twitter feeds:

www.theillustratednail.tumblr.com
www.sophiehg.virb.com
Instagram: @theillustratednail
Twitter: @illustratenail
YouTube: www.youtube.com/theillustratednail

SUPPLIERS, STOCKISTS & BRANDS

For polishes, and other essential nail tools and products in the UK and USA:

American Apparel: www.americanapparel.net
Barry M: www.barrym.com
Boots: www.boots.com
Color Club: www.colorclub.com
CVS: www.cvs.com
Elegant Touch: www.eleganttouch.com
MAC UK: www.maccosmetics.co.uk
MAC USA: www.maccosmetics.com
Madam Glam: www.madamglam.com
Mr. Nail Art (US only): www.mrnailart.com
    Instagram: @mrnailart
Nailene: www.nailene.com (Nailene Oval Full
    Cover Nails were used throughout the book)
Nails Supreme: www.nailssupremedesignernailart.com

The New Black: www.sephora.com/the-new-black
OPI UK: www.opiuk.com
OPI USA: www.opi.com
Revlon: www.revlon.com
Seche Vite: www.seche.com
Sephora: www.sephora.com
Sparkly Nails: www.sparkly-nails.co.uk
Superdrug: www.superdrug.com
Swarovski: http://crystals.swarovski.com/home/
    index.en.html
Topshop Beauty: www.topshop.com
Tweezerman USA: www.tweezerman.com
Tweezerman UK: www.tweezerman.co.uk